MAKING NICE WITH NAUGHTY

MAKING NICE WITH NAUGHTY

An Intimacy Guide for the Rule-Following, Organized, Perfectionist, Practical, and Color-Within-The-Line Types

THOMAS L. MURRAY, JR., PH. D.

ADVANCE PRAISE

"If you have been looking for a book that helps you and your partner understand how to let go of sexual perfectionism and start enjoying your sex life, *Making Nice with Naughty* is for you. In a kind but straightforward style, Dr. Tom Murray helps you identify why being in control and great sex don't make good bedfellows. Then you'll discover how to turn off that internal critical voice and express and receive the intimacy you really want."

Dr. Stephanie Buehler

Author, *What Every Mental Health Professional Needs to Know about Sex*, 3rd Ed.

"Dr. Murray reminds us why we often say that "the brain is the biggest sex organ." *Making Nice with Naughty* is a timely discussion on the connection between personality and sexuality. This book offers realistic examples of how our memories, thoughts, and the mind-body connection can impact our sex lives and relationships. This book can help enlighten anyone seeking answers to a possible void or challenge in their sex lives. If you are curious about yourself or others, this book provides valuable insights."

Tanya M. Bass, Ph.D., CHES®, CSE

The Southern Sexologist ™

"If you or someone you know can't put aside life's demands long enough to enjoy the simple pleasures of sex, then *Making Nice with Naughty* is the book for you. Through his personal, relatable, and thought-provoking writing style, Dr. Murray guides readers on how to tame the greatest obstacle to sexual enjoyment, themselves."

Samuel Sanabria, Ph.D., AASECT Certified Sex Therapist
Professor in Clinical Mental Health Counseling, Rollins College

"If your Over-Controlling Inner Assholes are ruining your intimate relationships, *Making Nice with Naughty* is your roadmap for letting go, enjoying the ride, and reconnecting to yourself and your partner(s)."

Lynn Dutrow, LCPC

Author, *ALIGNED As F*ck: Transforming Your Inner Assholes (like Anxiety) into Allies*

"A skillful blend of therapeutic knowledge, assertiveness, and compassion, Dr. Murray succinctly offers clear explanations palatable for the general public as well as for professionals. His clinical approach working with individuals and relationships comes through beautifully as if he's sitting right across from you."

Dr. Reece Malone - Sex Therapist & Sexuality Educator

Co-editor of *An Intersectional Approach to Sex Therapy*

COPYRIGHT

First published in 2022

by Clinical Training & Consultation, PLLC

612 N. Greene Street, Greensboro, NC 27401

Copyright© 2022 Thomas L. Murray, Jr., Ph.D.

The right of Thomas L. Murray, Jr. to be identified as the authors of this manuscript has been asserted in accordance with sections 77 and 78 of the Copyright, Designs and Patents Act 1988.

All rights reserved. No part of this book may be reproduced or reprinted in any form or by any means, electronic or mechanical, including photocopying, recording, or by any information storage and retrieval system, without permission in writing from the publisher.

Case studies used in this book are either fictional or information about individuals has been changed to protect their identity.

For permission to reprint material from this book, please visit

www.drtommurray.com.

Library of Congress Cataloging-in-Publication Data

Name: Murray, Jr, Thomas L.

Title: Making Nice with Naughty: An Intimacy Guide for the Rule-Following, Organized, Perfectionist, Practical, and Color-Within-The-Line Types Description: Greensboro, NC: Clinical Training & Consultation, PLLC | Includes bibliographical references.

Identifiers: LCC 2022915473 | ISBN 9780578271385 (pbk. : alk. paper)

DEDICATION

To every rule-following, organized, perfectionist, practical, and color-within-the-line type who ever yearned to overcome the psychological and relationship obstacles preventing them from making nice with naughty. May this book empower you to lean into the awkward, release perfectionism, express vulnerability, and, most of all, have fun in and out of the bedroom.

CONTENTS

Acknowledgments 1

Introduction 2

Chapter 1: Rules, Rules, Rules! 9

Chapter 2: Making Nice with Naughty... 29

Chapter 3: Let Go of My Ego 47

Chapter 4: Igniting Your Fire of Desire.. 67

Chapter 5: Do Your Eyes Light Up?... 87

Chapter 6: Letting Your Values Guide You..................................... 109

Chapter 7: Making Friends with Anxiety 131

Chapter 8: Taming the Monkey.. 155

Chapter 9: Victim to Victorious 178

Chapter 10: Committing to the Vision... 213

About the Author 229

References 230

ACKNOWLEDGMENTS

I am grateful to the many individuals and couples I've consulted over the 20 years as a marriage and family therapist. Their courage, wisdom, and trust in me have been a continuous inspiration.

I'm also very grateful for those in my personal life who've tolerated my overcontrolled tendencies. These include my sons, Evan and Bryce, and those who've dared to be with me romantically. Many thanks, too, to Kirstie for being a witness to my life, loving me unconditionally, and accepting my idiosyncrasies.

I wish to thank my writing coach, John Fayad, whose constant encouragement, insights, and patience with my neuroses led to the completion of this manuscript.

Francis Robbins, PMHNP, has been a constant friend and mentor who encouraged me repeatedly to get this manuscript out, as well as my business coach, Jill Beresford, faculty member of the Goldman Sachs 10,000 Small Businesses program who foresaw this book's impact.

I would also like to thank the many thought leaders, authors, mental health professionals, colleagues, professors, mentors, and coaches who've shaped my understanding of the human condition. Special consideration goes to Thomas Lynch, PhD; Byron Katie and *The Work*; Eckhart Tolle; the works of psychiatrists Patrick Thomas Malone, MD and Thomas Patrick Malone, MD; the work of Carl Whitaker, MD; and the work of Albert Ellis and the Albert Ellis Institute.

INTRODUCTION

In September of 2020, during the height of the global COVID pandemic, I transitioned my sex therapy practice to telehealth. During one of these early autumn sessions, I had a light-bulb moment while working with a couple who presented with a desire discrepancy: he wanted more sex, and she, well, couldn't care less. Before they got too far into their story, the thought arose that I bet I could predict with considerable accuracy the nature of this couple's sex life by asking just one question:

"Are you a 'BE CAREFUL!' parent? Or, are you a 'Have fun!' parent?"

Kids take risks. They're natural explorers and discoverers. They feed off of adventure when left to their own devices. Yet their enthusiasm for leaping over steps, swinging high, or running like lightning down a hill triggers anxiety in many parents. These parents can't help but command their children to "Be careful! You might hurt yourself." All they (or maybe you) see is the possible injuries, not to mention the disruptions to plans or, God forbid, the possibility that the neighbors will think you're an unfit parent.

Before the stroke of insight that led to this provocative question, I had been studying a relatively new and emerging psychotherapy called Radically Open Dialectical Behavior Therapy (RODBT), developed by psychologist Thomas Lynch, Ph.D. Unlike its more famous cousin, Dialectical Behavior Therapy (DBT), which focuses on symptoms associated with the under-controlled coping style, RODBT focused on the problems most associated with having too much self-control (i.e., overcontrolled).

The overcontrolled (OC) temperament is like other temperaments, such as introversion and extraversion. Neither is right nor wrong, good nor bad. Rather, OC denotes a way of being in the world. People who lean toward OC are likely to be the rule-following, organized, perfectionistic, practical, and color-within-the-line types. Sound familiar? I describe OC in much more detail in Chapter 1, which includes a self-test for gauging your degree of OC.

Jessica was one of these patients who had too much self-control. *"My mind just won't shut off, especially during sex,"* Jessica complained as we met over my telehealth platform. She and her husband, Chris, had been experiencing sexual problems for some time, which included growing emotional distance from each other. Their relationship satisfaction worsened as the years passed and their family grew. Now it's gotten to the point where Jessica and Chris are desperate for things to change. Each fear that not changing will bring about the death of their relationship, Yet they're desperate for answers to get through this predicament.

Jessica clarified how she felt. *"I'm just not interested in sex very much. Sure, it feels good when we have it, but I am totally fine without it. It's like my mind can't settle down. It immediately focuses on the never-ending to-do list or worries about whether it can all get done. I'm always stressed and can't help but think my time might be better spent elsewhere. Honestly, even when I do have time for sex, I'd rather sleep. It's sad to say, and I feel bad about it, but it's true."*

She described herself as someone who has always been highly ambitious. As she recalled, in middle school and high school, she didn't quite fit in with the other girls. They chased boys while she kept her nose to the grindstone, getting superior grades and attending various extracurricular activities. Jessica had no trouble delaying gratification to achieve her bigger goals. These traits made her attractive to Chris, too.

Nevertheless, she'd be the first to admit her successes weren't salve for her chronic feelings of inadequacy, loneliness, and social isolation. Sure, she had sexual feelings during adolescence and early adulthood, but she suppressed those feelings. The fear of pregnancy or contracting an STI was sufficient to put sex off until marriage. When she reached college, she chose to stay in an all-female dorm while many of her friends chose the co-ed options. She didn't want any temptations or complications.

In short, Jessica was all work and no play. Her to-do list took priority over her getting-done list. Moreover, Chris' requests for more sex made sex feel like it was just another chore to her. She told herself that she was having sex for his benefit. Sex had minimal appeal in the face of the other distractions.

Michael, a 30-something-year-old, saw me for a different set of problems. He described himself as socially awkward and a late bloomer. Unlike Jessica, he wanted to pursue sexual partners but felt too anxious about it, fearing he'd make a fool out of himself. He was tall and lanky and had a complex about it. While many describe Michael as attractive, he never felt like he measured up. Despite this, he had a few sexual partners, mostly one-night-stands. The tables turned when he met Marlena, a woman whom he had been dating for about a year. He told me, *"I knew this was different; I saw a future with Marlena. She made me feel comfortable."*

Unfortunately, several months before seeing me, Michael experienced an inability to get an erection after a night of drinking, which hadn't happened to him before. *"Do you realize how embarrassing it is to want to have sex when your dick doesn't work? It's mortifying!"* he exclaimed.

Michael expected an erection every time he wanted one. It had been the case before when he mixed alcohol with sex; why should this be any different? The erectile issue flooded him with anxiety and made him question his masculinity, as well as wrestle with the question of whether Marlena had judged him. He described how he had begun pulling away from Marlena, fearing she would want sex and he'd experience a repeat of his mortifying event.

In their own distinct relationships. Michael and Jessica suffer from sexual perfectionism—a common attribute among OCs. Sexual perfectionism has various types but includes one or more of the following beliefs: (1) I have to be sexually perfect, (2) my partner has to be sexually perfect, (3) I think my partner thinks I have to be sexually perfect, and (4) society expects me to be sexually perfect. You can see through the above scenarios that Jessica and Michael believe certain conditions must be met to enjoy sex. If the conditions are absent, this provokes feelings of uncertainty and vulnerability, both major impediments to sexual enjoyment for OC people. For Jessica, sexual readiness includes the completion of a never-ending to-do list. On the other hand, Michael believes that his penis should become erect on demand just because he wants it to. In short, both have become psychologically rigid and rule-based regarding their sexuality in maladaptive ways.

Perhaps you found yourself connecting with some or all of Jessica's and Michael's stories. However, your feeling of familiarity with their story may not be enough to convince you that this book is relevant to your life. I get it.

As I've mentioned before, you don't like uncertainty. It makes total sense that you want to know immediately whether this book is for you. You don't have time or money to waste. It's like that vacuum you bought several years ago. Remember? You spent weeks researching the options, including studying *Consumer Reports* to ensure that you wouldn't eventually regret your decision. You don't like to feel disappointed and, indeed, you hate surprises, especially those that could lead to regret.

Hopefully, when you picked up this book, you saw yourself in the subtitle. You immediately connected the part of you that recognized something missing within your sex and intimate relationship and the aspect of your personality that struggles with having fun, especially in the bedroom.

This book is written specifically for you: someone who's taken life too seriously, who has high personal standards, and regularly sacrifices your personal needs to get that next promotion, professional award, or personal achievement.

In your hands is an intimacy guide for turning down the dial on your overcontrolled temperament and reclaiming psychological flexibility, child-like playfulness, adventure, and guilt-free pleasure-seeking. However, this book isn't a promise to rid yourself of anxiety. Nor is this book about curing you of your overcontrolled tendencies. There's nothing inherently wrong with being overcontrolled. I'm overcontrolled, and I like many of these facets of my personality. However, I recognized that this too-much-of-a-good-thing could negatively impact people's sex lives and intimate relationships.

On this journey with me, you and I will honor those parts working well for you while minimizing the negative impact this coping style has on your pursuit of a meaningful and fulfilling relationship. In a moment, I'll provide you with a high-level summary of each chapter. Take a moment and review what's in store. No surprises!

But before we begin, let me bring your attention to the concept of *Psychological Obesity*. This occurs due to the regular consumption of thoughts and ideas that aren't metabolized into action. It's just as if you were to eat too many calories for your needs, you'll gain weight. Likewise, OCs tend to consume many ideas by reading self-help books, listening to podcasts, and on and on, hoping to find the perfect answers that ensure they'll avoid problems in the future. However, action means uncertainty in the outcome. Consequently, OCs can find that they often don't take action despite having excellent ideas. Let's not make that happen here.

I don't want you just to read this book and move on to the next self-help author. This is not just a book of ideas. Sure, I want you to learn more about yourself and your psychology (I'm a shrink; I get off on that shit!). But more importantly, I want you to develop psychological flexibility, identify what's really important, and take committed action toward your values. I'll ask that you experiment with life more than you've ever done before, which includes changing your relationship with certain feelings, such as anxiety, awkwardness, and uncertainty. To that end, here are the insights you will gain in each chapter.

In **Chapter 1**, I'll introduce you to the four key traits of an overcontrolled temperament, the high cost of having too much self-control in the context of making nice with naughty, and where you may lie on the overcontrolled/under-controlled continuum.

Chapter 2 makes the connection of your OC temperament to your struggles with sexuality and intimacy in your relationships. Those same admirable qualities that have and continue to serve you well in other areas of your life may be posing challenges for you in the bedroom and in establishing and maintaining long-term intimate relationships.

In **Chapter 3**, I explain how your ego, the continuous mind chatter that tries to narrate of your life isn't the real you. The great truth is that you are not your experience but rather the observer of your experience. You'll discover why any hope of making nice with naughty begins with embracing the real you from this higher perspective.

Regaining lost intimacy and desire is the most coveted request of couples attracted to my practice. In **Chapter 4**, you'll discover why reigniting sexual desire in your relationships requires (1) fuel, the small, everyday contributions to the relationship, and (2) oxygen, the embodied view of yourself as a sexual being deserving of sexual expression and fulfillment, free of anxiety and fear.

Chapter 5 illustrates how the OC trait of a neutral face and constraining emotional expression to veil feelings of vulnerability or conceal emotions can work to your advantage at funerals and business meetings, yet be misconstrued as threatening, stand-offish, and aloof when it comes to intimate relationships.

In **Chapter 6**, I applied the concept of values to the context of making nice with naughty to help you clarify what's important to you

Making Nice with Naughty

vis-à-vis your sexual behavior. I invite you to examine whether your sexual and intimate behaviors reflect your values and serve as guideposts for living an authentic life.

Chapter 7 provides a framework to help change your relationship with anxiety and learn to live with it—even draw strength from it—by creating an "optimum balance" that reclaims your innate sexual self. You'll learn strategies to support your new reasoning by disputing irrational beliefs and experiencing the positive effect healthier thoughts can have on your sex life.

Chapter 8 then offers a series of mindfulness meditations designed to help turn down the volume on your mind chatter and bring you closer to the optimum balance you'll have discovered within yourself. Even if a novice to meditation, you'll learn methods for developing greater mindfulness to turn down the dial, not off, on your OC temperament and tame the dancing monkey inside your head.

This book wouldn't be complete if I didn't devote a chapter to those who have experienced sexual trauma in their lives and how their experience intersects with the value of making nice with naughty. In **Chapter 9**, you'll learn how the story we tell ourselves about our trauma is the biggest impediment to finding enjoyment and fulfillment in our sexual life and intimate relationships. You'll also learn how and why forgiveness, as an act of self-love, can be an essential part of your ability to grow from victim to victorious and reclaim, or claim for the first time in your life, yourself as a sexual being.

Each chapter contains exercises that I use in my practice to help deepen your learning, unearth rational reasoning, dispute your irrational beliefs, and migrate you from a fixed or fatalistic mindset to one of openness and possibility. In this book, you will find the path to co-existing with your anxieties and fears.

Okay. That's enough jibber-jabber. Let's start your journey toward making nice with naughty.

CHAPTER 1
RULES, RULES, RULES!

"Don't be careful, you could hurt yourself."

— Byron Katie

You've perfected self-control. Your whole life has been about delaying gratification, inhibiting your impulses, and suppressing your desires. In fact, you were likely the trusted kid your parents knew would never throw a party if they went away for the weekend. Sure, you might have thought about it, but you'd quickly remind yourself of all that could go wrong if you got caught: friends wrecking the place, drugs and alcohol everywhere, and neighbors calling the police! You were taught that being naughty was dangerous and rife with consequences; you wanted to be good and be admired by important people in your life.

The lesson of childhood was that self-control was the royal road to excellence. You were highly rewarded for your ability to suspend your enjoyment of even the most minor things to achieve your goals. Perhaps your family equated success with happiness; and since middle school, you were reminded of the importance of planning and preparation as essential ingredients for winning. The game was about anticipating problems and strategizing how to overcome them. And while you likely excelled at academics, you were anxious about making mistakes and plagued by questions of whether you were good enough.

I remember my middle and high school years, recalling each of the moments, even the content of conversations, that exposed my overcontrolled tendencies as a teen. I recollect riding the school bus one morning with my friend Sam during which I shared my weekend adventures. Sam interjected, *"Why don't you act your age?"*

Typically, that remark signals disapproval for a person acting beneath their age. Not in my case; I was the exact opposite! I was a 40-year-old trapped in a 15-year-old's body. There was a clear seriousness in how I lived life. In short, I was hyper-mature, a common trait of many young, overcontrolled people. Raise your hand if you were ever told that you were an "old soul." Yep, there you are! I certainly heard it many times.

This isn't to say that I was straight-laced 100 percent of the time. Many friends and family experienced me as the life of the party. Others experienced me as a pain in the ass, too. Don't let me kid you. I was the class clown and certainly not timid. However, people didn't realize that much thought went into my social interactions, including the timing and delivery of jokes. I was serious about my fun, unable to fully relax in the company of others or thoroughly cut loose when everyone around me was having fun. If they were having "too much fun," I became nervous, tense, and worried that friends would embarrass themselves or, worse yet, embarrass me. I couldn't bear others thinking poorly of me, even if by association. These social situations would often leave me feeling powerless.

Perhaps like me, from an early age your definition of success was characterized by acquiring a sense of safety and security—your barometers for a well-lived life. Your routines meant sacrificing and saying no to your friends because of commitments and obligations. You didn't waste any time getting home from school each day to practice the piano or violin, rehearse at the dance studio or practice on the field, or clean your room and be around if your parents needed you. You might have noticed that your close friends seldom extended invitations to you anymore because they figured you once again say,

"I'm too busy." All the while, you may also have had the feeling of not quite belonging; somehow you were an outsider.

Nevertheless, you found your efforts paid off later in life. Your employers love you and get you stellar performance reviews year after year. You're not afraid of hard work. You show up early and stay late, and you're willing to work weekends if necessary. You're prized for your attention to detail and consistently meeting deadlines or achieving quotas. You're always ready, available, and willing to get the job done, and have done exceptionally well. Some may have even thrown the "workaholic" label at you from time to time. On the other hand, your colleagues and those you supervise might report being intimidated by you, your productivity, and your stick-to-itiveness. You, however, simply describe yourself as committed, loyal, and dedicated to doing a good job and getting that next promotion.

Undoubtedly, the industrious and productive behaviors of OC people are highly praised in societies around the world, as is their resistance to the temptation of immediate pleasure in the hope of obtaining a valuable and long-lasting reward. Many cultures, religions, and philosophies value delayed gratification as one of the highest human virtues. We teach our children to admire and emulate those who show self-restraint, compliance, and sacrifice. We punish and look down upon those who are disruptive, impulsive, distracted, and unpredictable.

No one tells us, nor do we learn from experience, that there are high costs in having too much self-control (i.e., self-regulation). Sure, there's virtue in sacrificing a little personal gratification now and again, but for some, sacrificing can become *again* and *again* and *again*. An overcontrolled temperament (i.e., too much self-control) can become one's way of life and, for many, lead to the following:

- an increased sense of loneliness

- interpersonal problems, particularly within romantic and familial relationships
- over-the-top perfectionism, including sexual perfectionism
- difficulty taking risks
- not having the flexibility and adaptability required to adjust to the unpredictability of life

Are you overcontrolled? Do the descriptions and stories that I've shared with you thus far ring true? Have I touched on something you've often wondered about yourself or just accepted as your personality type? Perhaps it never fully dawned on you that too much self-control was possible, that it carried such cost, or that there would be any reason to change.

Too Much of a Good Thing

Temperament is an aspect of your personality concerned with emotional tendencies and reactions. They represent personality traits that are stable over time. For example, extroversion and introversion are well-known personality temperaments and fall on a continuum from extraverted to introverted. Another temperament that lies on a continuum, which is the focus of my book, is the under-controlled (UC) and overcontrolled (OC) temperament.

On one end of the spectrum, we have UC people characterized as open, mood-oriented, unstructured, and uninhibited. On the other hand, OC people are rule-oriented, structured, and risk-averse. It's important to say that, just as with extroversion and introversion, your place on the UC/OC continuum is neither right nor wrong, good nor bad. Both temperaments have their strengths and limitations depending on the context in which they're expressed. In short, temperament describes aspects of your personality and how you show up in the world.

OC people, myself included, usually have great pride around our capacity to be highly self-controlled, which is why overcontrolled is often characterized as the "too-much-of-a-good-thing" syndrome (i.e., we value and hold in high esteem those who are disciplined and have high personal standards). We admire people who pursue accuracy, work hard, sacrifice for their families, and contribute to the good of society.

However, when you're too overcontrolled, you may find that particular disposition can interfere with the parts of your life that require adaptability, flexibility, and enjoyment. As a result, many OC people experience suppressed sexuality and problems within intimate relationships, two topics discussed in more detail in the pages to come.

Many overcontrolled, rule-driven factors can suppress sexuality for both men and women. For example, many overcontrolled men share a common apprehension: the fear of offending someone by commenting on their attractiveness or tripping over their words and saying something socially stupid. They'll hesitate to pursue someone sexually or romantically for fear of being seen as a creep or desperate. OC men can be apprehensive in leaning in for a kiss on the first date for fear of being rebuffed. Some OC heterosexual men, with their hyper-focus on respecting boundaries, are misperceived as gay by the women they're with because they tend not to flirt or make any moves on the first date.

Many rules for OC men suppress sexual expression and inhibit sexual satisfaction. A big one for guys (no pun intended) is having a mindset filled with rules and anxieties about getting an erection at the right time and maintaining it as long as possible. Another rule is when to orgasm or whether it's their responsibility to bring their partner to orgasm. Excuse me, but if those are the rules running through your head instead of how beautiful that moment is, you'll get pumped up with adrenaline, get buried in the details, lose your hard-on, and ejaculate too soon or not at all. Consequently, OC men are susceptible to premature ejaculation, delayed ejaculation, low sexual desire, and/or sexual shame around fetishes or other sexual interests.

OC women also have rules that interfere with their sexual enjoyment and expression as sexual beings. For example, a common rule is the "I must feel connected first to have sex." They may feel horny but don't pursue sexual pleasure because of a perceived absence of connection or lingering resentment. In general, OC people tend to be highly moralistic and have strong beliefs about how the world *"should be, must be, or has to be."* They can be very principled about what's right and wrong, and if something feels wrong, they will not pursue their sexual pleasure if it were to inadvertently reinforce their partner's bad behavior.

Overcontrolled women can also have difficulty reaching orgasm, even with direct clitoral stimulation. Why? Because, like OC men, they get into their heads, unable to relax and focus on the beautiful moment at hand. OC women can experience anxiety from mind chatter about a conflict at work or at home, whether the kids will walk into the room, if the front door is locked, or if the oven's off. Like men, OC women can struggle with how to be fully present during sexual intimacy (or anything that requires present-moment awareness).

Moreover, some OC women experience sexual pain due to vaginismus—a tightening of the muscles surrounding the vaginal canal. It's the body's automatic reaction to the fear of vaginal penetration, making penetration painful. As you can imagine, all of these various factors make sex stressful, and with stress, sex becomes less desirable.

Why You're Here

Many reasons drew you to this book, but you connected with the book's title and description for a reason. You're here because you're feeling something missing in your sex life. You want to live life fully, and you innately know that sexual health is an essential part of your experience of being human. In short, you want to reduce sexual inhibitions and find ways to make nice with naughty.

Why you're here is why my patients come to me: they're anxious and depressed about their sex life—a sex life where they feel sexually blocked, self-conscious, and sexually constrained. Like many of my patients, you want to claim your right to sexual pleasure and fulfillment. I also share your story.

Soon after my former partner and I separated, I found a psychologist and met with her weekly. It was early in our sessions, the first or second, I think, when I said to her, *"You know, I've come to realize that I don't exude much of a sexuality."*

She let the declaration sit for a moment, looked me in the eyes, and said, *"Tom, you're right; you don't."*

Some might say that my psychologist's response was harsh and blunt, but it was exactly what I needed to hear. I spent much of that relationship trying to be an excellent partner and often failing to the point of suppressing my sexuality. I subconsciously believed I didn't deserve the sexual desires that would eventually become dormant; I simply buried them. What I know now, however, is that when we bury our feelings, we bury them alive, which is especially true for sexual energy.

Feelings of being sexually bottled up are why you're here. Parts of you want to be free. Or, perhaps, your partner has become resentful and complained that they want more sex than you. On the surface, you agree with them, but not for the reasons they think; you know there's something more at play. It's that innate understanding that you've been missing out that drove you to pick up this book—a knowing that sexuality is an integral, meaningful part of your life and your partner's life.

You're also here because you're deeply aware that your intimate relationship suffers. You excel in many areas, but a lasting, meaningful, and fulfilling intimate relationship eludes you. You've lost the sex drive you once had. You're often frustrated in your ability to express yourself sexually, perhaps even afraid. You might struggle to help your partner express themselves fully so they can find satisfaction. You want to become more spontaneous, but something is holding you back. You want to find out what that something is and make nice with it so you'll again, or for the first time, be able to express and find enjoyment in your sexuality.

Just as I tell my patients, I don't profess to have a prescription that will cure your overcontrolled temperament. In fact, there are not enough drugs or therapy in the world that will make me under-controlled, and it may be that way for you. Besides, I don't want to be under-controlled; I like who I am and what I've accomplished. Nevertheless, I've worked to identify contexts (namely, intimate and sexual relationships) where I can turn down my overcontrolledness to get more of what I want. I trust that you'll also benefit from my personal and professional experiences. My book offers a context for understanding your overcontrolled temperament and helping you make sense of it so that you can get to the nub of why you have the experiences you're having.

But don't just trust me; trust your observations of your behaviors and experiences compared with the common traits of OC people and the real-life stories of patients described throughout my book. Of course, their names and details have been changed, but their experiences with the world around them are authentic—and you may discover that their experiences resonate with your own. Let's further deepen the dive into the characteristics of an overcontrolled temperament.

The Four Traits of an Overcontrolled Person

As you've probably gathered from the stories and examples of the behaviors of OC people, there are many in the world, and they can be anyone. I'm one, and you might be one as well. It's all a matter of degree; some lean slightly OC while others lean quite far into the OC trait. Depending on where you are on the continuum will determine the intensity of your behavior. When one's OC level moves from adaptive or productive, where self-control is a strength and a virtue, to an OC level that's maladaptive or nonproductive, problems arise, particularly within sex and intimate relationships.

In some regions of our lives, as in our careers, self-control is a highly prized personality trait. Employers, friends, and colleagues, for example, find us immensely dependable, driven, dedicated, committed, detail-oriented, persistent, and loyal. All virtues, right? However, often these traits hide underlying insecurities, especially around vulnerability and the fear of losing or being out of control.

In the context of an intimate relationship where sex should be about fun, playfulness, mystery, and exploration, you need to be able to dial down the volume on your OC tendencies so that you can tap into the power of social connections and vulnerability for more enjoyable sexual experiences and intimate relationships. If you fit the bill on the traits of an OC person that I'm about to share and want meaning and purpose in your sex life, you're going to have to do something different because what you've been doing thus far is not working for you, and possibly not for your partner as well.

Thomas R. Lynch is an American psychologist, author, and treatment developer of Radically Open Dialectical Behavior Therapy (RODBT), a type of psychotherapy that targets psychiatric disorders characterized by excessive self-control (e.g., anorexia, Obsessive-Compulsive Personality Disorder, Autism Spectrum, treatment-resistant anxiety and depression, maladaptive perfectionism). Lynch's identification and categorization of OC traits provide a thoughtful and comprehensive model for describing an overcontrolled personality.[1]

---

[1] Lynch, Thomas R., PhD FBPsS (February 15, 2018). *Radically Open Dialectical Behavior Therapy: Theory and Practice for Treating Disorders of Overcontrol*, pp 7–18. Context Press.

This book applies Lynch's research, which I integrated with works from other thought leaders, to address the sexual and relationship struggles of so many OCs. Let's begin your journey of self-discovery by completing Lynch's *Style of Coping* assessment[2] at the end of this chapter. The *Styles of Coping* assessment features 47 word-pairs that will help you determine whether you lean under-controlled or overcontrolled.

Lynch developed four categories that portray a grouping of characteristics or dimensions of an OC person: (1) low receptivity and openness to the unexpected; (2) inflexibility and hyper-perfectionism; (3) expressionlessness and unawareness; and (4) undeveloped interpersonal dynamics. Let's look into the elements of each and, through example, how each characteristic shows itself in our lives and our relationships.

1. Low Receptivity and Openness to the Unexpected

This first trait of an OC person is reflected in their struggle with being open to new or unexpected situations. The OC temperament can get in the way of receiving important feedback about yourself, your openness and flexibility to respond to new situations, and maintaining meaningful and fulfilling intimate relationships. Novel situations are risky, and OC people are risk-averse and hypervigilant to any potential threats in their environment. They back away from whatever triggers a sense of vulnerability. They'll avoid unplanned events or exposure to invalidating situations that don't align with their beliefs or how things should be done.

Retrieved from https://www.amazon.com/Radically-Open-Dialectical-Behavior-Therapy/dp/1626259283?asin=1626259283&revisionId=&format=4&depth=1

[2] Ibid, Appendix 1: Assessing Styles of Coping Word-Pair Checklist.

It's Thursday, and your partner was invited to an impromptu party Friday evening by a friend at work. Your partner comes home and shares the exciting news that you're invited, too. What is your typical and immediate reaction? Do you say, *"No,"* and come up with excuses about how tired you are or how you don't want to drive anymore for the day?

You're not alone on this one. Saying no first is a very common overcontrolled response. OC people are typically not open to unexpected events that are not on their schedule or don't fit their rules, which means informing you at least a few days in advance that there will be a party—not the day before. You had nothing planned that evening and could have easily gone, but you don't like surprises, and now neither of you is going.

Such rules aren't limited to mundane invitations. Rules can surround even more momentous occasions. Brenda and Kevin dated for several months. One evening, they began talking about marriage. Brenda was particularly insistent that they get married because they were living together. Kevin loved Brenda and wanted to marry her, but Brenda hated surprises. She was clear that she wanted advanced notice of any proposal. Kevin reluctantly obliged. He got the ring several weeks later and awkwardly announced to Brenda, *"Let's go to the mountains this weekend so I can propose."* No surprises, right? Nor is it remotely romantic.

Another indicator of low receptivity and low openness in OC people is their high sensitivity to eliminating threats to their comfort, safety, and security. This is often fueled by fears of vulnerability where they'll be exposed and feel insecure. An unplanned event fits their definition of a potential threat because it's risky and creates uncertainty. It can show itself in many ways that go unnoticed. OC people will frequent the same restaurant, for example, and order the same thing, rationalizing, *"Well, I know what I like; why risk going to a place that could serve me something I won't like?"*

The third dimension of this trait is the tendency to discount or dismiss critical feedback or any form of constructive criticism. OC people find it difficult to receive feedback in general, chiefly because everyone around them perceives them as highly competent and highly effective, as many OCs are. Multiply that by their perception of themselves as rarely being wrong. The idea of negative feedback becomes incongruous with their view of themselves and is straightaway discounted and ignored. However, it's a thin shell covering their feelings of vulnerability.

Criticism, even advice, triggers the OC person's perpetual sense of underachieving and heightens their unending feelings of not measuring up. Even someone disagreeing with what they're saying in a friendly conversation has the potential to fuel their anxiety and cause them to feel exposed and unprotected. Consequently, OC people may withdraw emotionally or physically in the face of critical feedback.

2. Inflexible and Hyper-Perfectionist

This side of an OC person expresses a compulsive need for structure, order, and rules for regulating themselves and the anxiety that arises out of uncertainty, unpredictability, and perceived chaos. OC people possess a very high work ethic and display a deep social obligation as well as having a sense of duty in bringing organization to things.

They often describe themselves as perfectionists, but others might say they're more hyper-perfectionist with their compulsive planning, rehearsing, and correcting. Their lives are guided by rigid rules that govern their behavior, and their high moral certainty is fueled by their conviction that there is one "right" way to do something. A classic example is going behind your partner to rearrange the dishwasher because they didn't do it right. (I know who you are; I do it, too!) You might ask that others not do your laundry because you want to ensure that it's washed and folded correctly.

Another feature of OCs is their emphasis on clock time. They find great comfort in their schedule where the clock determines the start and stop of activities rather than their personal needs. For example, John won't eat lunch until noon. It's his rule. Although his body tells him, *"Hey, John, I'm hungry; I need to eat something,"* if it's not the right time, that is, if the clock on the wall doesn't read twelve-zero-zero, then the body is going to have to wait.

Likewise, sex can become regimented where there's a defined time when sex can happen; if it doesn't happen during that time, then it's not going to happen at all. In essence, OC folks find great comfort and security in conforming to an external standard that they've established; if an activity or behavior doesn't fit within that standard, they won't satisfy that desire. In essence, they dissociate from their bodies and rely on an external measure to govern their behavior.

When it comes to hyper-perfectionism, there are people you probably know (I certainly do) who are never wrong about anything. When you think about it, they are seldom wrong about things, given the intense amount of time they spend researching and reflecting on the details of something important to them.

The same three couples have taken a week-long vacation every year on the Florida Gulf Coast for the past twenty years. And every year, Judy gets very tense about her beach time and having her giant umbrellas perfectly distanced from the ocean. She studies the tides every day to know exactly where to have her husband pitch the umbrellas at 11:00 AM so that by 4:00 PM when they leave, the incoming tide is a comfortable distance away. The other couples benefit from Judy's hyper-perfectionism by simply pitching their umbrellas alongside hers, which inadvertently accommodates her anxiety.

OC people are often correct about things. They've done the research and fixated on details I wouldn't have. The problem for Judy and those like her, though, is that the enjoyment of the activity can get lost among the strict adherence to rules. For example, Judy will spend five hours of beach time each day, which she longs for all year long, concerning herself with people pitching their umbrellas in front of hers and blocking her view of the ocean. The strict adherence to the rules about how things should or must go keeps her from thoroughly enjoying the time at the beach with friends.

3. Emotionally Expressionless and Unaware

This characteristic of OC people centers on social cues, the verbal and non-verbal signals we express primarily through our face, body, and voice. These signals guide our interactions with others and influence how we respond to them.

By and large, OC people's social signaling is tempered, and they tend to show restricted facial expressions. If a friend runs up and screams that she just won a million dollars in the lottery, an overcontrolled person would calmly and collectedly say, *"Oh, that's great. How are you going to spend the money?"* On the other hand, an under-controlled person would most likely start screaming and jumping up and down with excitement for your windfall.

Two stories stand out for me related to my lack of facial expression. A college professor reviewed my videotapes when I trained to become a psychotherapist. He said, *"Tom, you have really perfected the poker face."* He then said, *"The problem with the poker face is that the client ultimately is left feeling insecure and wondering what you're doing with the information they're giving you."*

That observation of my overcontrolled tendencies was no different from Sam's on the school bus 30 years ago, telling me that I wasn't acting my age.

Later, after having practiced for several years, I sat with a patient who suddenly exclaimed, *"Sometimes, when you look at me, I have the sense that at any given moment you're going to pull a knife from behind your back and eviscerate me."* Somewhat startled, the only thing that I could think of to say was, *"So, you're afraid that I might make you spill your guts."* Clearly channeling my inner Freud in that moment!

Pay an OC person a compliment, and their temperament often prevents them from responding with an authentic smile and genuine expression of thanks. Conversely, they might execute a smile and acknowledge the compliment while silently doubting the validity of the praise. OCs will reserve expressing vulnerable emotions in private. For example, they'll cry during a movie when they're alone, but they'll suppress any emotional response if someone is with them, particularly someone who holds social capital. If an OC person is anxious or depressed, you wouldn't know it. Ask them how they feel or how they're doing, and you'll hear one of their favorite f-words, *"Fine."*

4. Undeveloped Interpersonal Dynamics

Someone aloof is not a person you'd consider warm and engaging. Instead, they're found to be distant and reserved. This third trait of OC people describes their tendency towards low social connectedness and intimacy with others. They're reluctant to start up conversations and can feel uncomfortable and self-conscious around others.

Emotional detachment is an inability or unwillingness to connect with others emotionally and often physically. OC people tend to feel awkward standing close to others, hugging, or holding hands. For some people, being emotionally detached helps protect them from unwanted drama, anxiety, or stress. It also minimizes their feelings of vulnerability.

This side of OC people includes their perception of themselves as different from everyone else. We tend to make many social comparisons on whether we measure up to our colleagues and friends. We can be envious of and bitter toward others and their successes, especially if their accomplishments directly impact our achievements.

By extension, overcontrolled people don't want to share a lot about themselves because the more they do, the more they could be judged.

OC people hold their cards close to their chest to avoid feeling exposed or giving someone something judgmental about them that could potentially diminish their social status.

An interesting aspect of this trait is that OC people may appear aloof and distant to everyone around them; yet internally they're hypervigilant and anxious, always in an elevated state of constantly assessing potential threats, especially when they're in the company of others. It's similar to a duck gliding along, appearing calm and collected on the surface while paddling like hell underneath.

I recall being proud that I never cried in any of my graduate classes. You might be thinking, *"Tom, why would you cry in graduate school anyway?"* Well, it's very common when you're in a mental health discipline because you're constantly exploring emotions, and your colleagues and friends are sharing poignant stories of themselves or friends and family. Classmates would cry when moved; it wasn't viewed as a weakness. I, on the other hand, suppressed my emotion and maintained an expressionless face. I was empathic towards my colleagues while feeling proud of being detached, not exposing my vulnerability, and acting professionally.

I think, on some level, I feared being judged or seen as weak if I showed emotion. I know I'm not alone in this fear. Humans want to feel as if we belong, that we are part of a tribe; consequently, we avoid doing anything that could get us kicked out of the community. This fear of rejection has developed over millennia. Naturally, you and I proceed with caution within interpersonal relationships to reduce the risk of judgments that would lead to being booted out. However, when it comes to strengthening social bonds (particularly romantic bonds), vulnerability, physical contact, and affection (e.g., hand-holding, hugging) are vital; they nurture a meaningful sexual and intimate relationship.

I ended up not making it through my entire graduate school without crying. It snuck up on me during one of my final classes when

I shared a childhood memory involving my relationship with my father. Suddenly, I welled up with tears and lost my composure. Lynch labels this phenomenon *emotional leakage,* the sudden and intense release of emotion that wouldn't normally be expressed in social situations. Emotional leakage can relate to an array of emotions: anger, sadness, anxiety, etc. At any rate, what I learned from my experience was that my tears, though causing me to feel embarrassed, made others feel closer to me and promoted social bonding.

"Where Do You Want to Go?"

What does a taxi driver say when you first get in her cab? *"Where do you want to go?"* She's not interested in where you've been. Nor does she care about your childhood and what your home life was like growing up. She wants to know where you're headed, and she promises to facilitate getting you there.

This metaphor defines my style of therapy and the value of my book to you. Your sex life is either moving you in the direction you want to go, or it's not. That's the only reality we're going to deal with. I'm interested and supportive of where you want to be in making nice with naughty in your relationship.

Overcontrolled temperament contributes to people's dissatisfaction in their sex life, perhaps in yours as well. You realize that something is missing, maybe now that the kids are grown and gone, or you and your partner are drifting apart, or your search for someone has been less than fulfilling. In the pages that follow, I provide a process for rekindling desire and bringing more meaning and fulfillment to your sex life.

Like a cabbie, I'm not interested in why you got to where you are today—ruminating on the why hasn't worked. For you, the *"why"* is less important than the *"what"* you will do now. Perhaps you're learning for the first time that an overcontrolled temperament is a definable thing and that it is most likely associated with sexual suppression and inhibited sexual satisfaction. You want to do something about it, and you're going to discover that you can.

Now that you paid the taxi fare in buying my book, where do you want to go with your sex life? My hope for you is that in the chapters to follow, the information, stories, and methodologies that I'll be sharing will help you identify and overcome the obstacles that keep you from expressing and finding enjoyment in your sexuality—that is, making nice with naughty.

Before we dive into Chapter 2 and the ways an overcontrolled temperament can affect sexual relationships and your ability to feel comfortable making nice with naughty, take the "Style of Coping" test developed by Dr. Thomas Lynch at the end of this chapter to help you determine where you lie on the UC/OC continuum.

Thomas L. Murray, Jr., Ph.D.

EXERCISE: STYLE OF COPING WORD-PAIRS

Read each word-pair in each row and place a check mark next to the word that best describes you. If you are unsure which word fits best, imagine what your friends or family members might say about you. If neither of the terms describes you—pick the one that is the closest to how you would describe yourself. Make sure that you choose only one word or phrase in each row.

This scale measures overall personality styles. A high score on either subscale does not necessarily indicate maladaptive under-controlled or overcontrolled coping. As with extroverted and introverted behavior, neither is right nor wrong. The scale simply describes your personality and how you show up in the world.

Impulsive		Deliberate	
Impractical		Practical	
Naive		Worldly	
Vulnerable		Aloof	
Risky		Prudent	
Talkative		Quiet	
Disobedient		Dutiful	
Fanciful		Realistic	
Fickle		Constant	
Act without Thinking		Think before acting	
Animated		Restrained	
Changeable Mood		Stable Mood	
Haphazard		Orderly	
Wasteful		Frugal	
Affable		Reserved	
Impressionable		Not easily impressed	
Erratic		Predictable	
Complaining		Uncomplaining	
Reactive		Unreactive	
Careless		Fastidious	
Playful		Earnest	

Intoxicated			Clear-headed		
Self-indulgent			Self-controlled		
Laid Back			Hard-working		
Unconventional			Conventional		
Dramatic			Modest		
Brash			Unobtrusive		
Obvious			Discreet		
Vacillating			Determined		
Unrealistic			Sensible		
Gullible			Shrewd		
Unpredictable			Dependable		
Dependent			Independent		
Improper			Proper		
Chaotic			Organized		
Susceptible			Impervious		
Unstable			Steadfast		
Volatile			Undemonstrative		
Excitable			Stoical		
Lax			Precise		
Unsystematic			Structured		
Thoughtless			Thoughtful		
Inattentive			Attentive		
Short-lived			Enduring		
Perky			Despondent		
Passionate			Indifferent		
Immediate gratification			Delay gratification		
Total score A			**Total score B**		

Printed with permission from New Harbinger Publications, Inc.

Tally up the number of checks in each column to determine your score. The column with the greatest number represents your overall coping style. If you have a higher score for column A, you tend to be more under-controlled. If you have a higher score for column B, you tend to be more overcontrolled.

CHAPTER 2
MAKING NICE WITH NAUGHTY

"When I'm good, I'm very good; but when I'm bad, I'm better."

— Mae West

Carl grew up in a family where high standards reigned supreme (e.g., only A's were acceptable; rigid rules around polite behavior; strict adherence to a piano practice schedule). From an early age, the young boy understood that he must meet others' expectations to make it in the world. The message was clear: others' opinions mattered. Consequently, whenever Carl stepped out of line, he got the message that he was naughty and good things don't happen to naughty boys. Good kids color within the lines. Good kids follow the rules and listen to authority. Good kids don't disrupt or interrupt. Good kids don't upset others. Good kids do what they're told. Mistakes were evidence of failure, and failure was unacceptable.

These factors, including his biology, contributed to Carl developing an overcontrolled temperament. He was domesticated to demand high expectations of himself. His pursuit of perfectionism drove him to do very well in almost all aspects of his life, from his scholastic achievements and a promising career with financial security to a meaningful and sexually active relationship.

Several weeks ago, Carl's sexual confidence began to unravel when he couldn't get an erection with his girlfriend, Maxine. Up until now, Carl took comfort in having predictable and consistently perfect erections. This night, though, was different. Maxine began to get intimate, but he noticed his dick wasn't getting hard, which freaked him out. He felt confused: he was turned on, but his dick wasn't showing up for the party. *"What the fuck?"* he thought.

His mind raced with anxious thoughts, and he couldn't relax and quiet his internal chatter. *"Men are supposed to be ready anytime! What if she thinks I'm not into her?"* Unfortunately, the only action he was getting that evening was the adrenaline pumping through his veins. (Little did he know, adrenaline inhibits genital response in both men and women.)

Carl was unable to relax and enjoy himself. Instead, he lay there overwhelmed with shame and embarrassment. Unfortunately, Maxine noticed as well. She tried to tell him that it was okay, but he could tell she was disappointed. Carl's problems persisted for several more weeks, and, consequently, his uncooperative penis triggered Maxine's anxiety about her attractiveness. Like so many women, she was taught that a man's erection signaled her worth and desirability. She began to resent Carl and even speculated whether he was gay.

Carl's feelings of embarrassment and shame intensified. He began to withdraw from Maxine, avoiding physical contact for fear that it might escalate into something sexual and he would fail again. He turned to porn and masturbation to prevent the possibility of future humiliation, which alienated Maxine even more. Maxine subsequently became concerned that Carl had developed a porn addiction. He hadn't; he simply couldn't manage the vulnerability that he felt in the face of his erectile problems.

Like so many men in this situation, Carl presumed he had a biological problem and pursued erectile dysfunction (ED) medication. He wanted to be confident that he could get an erection every time. Carl first met with a urologist who determined quickly that Carl's plumbing worked; it wasn't a medical issue. Consequently, Carl was given a referral to see me. When we met, we discussed what was happening. He said that he never had a problem getting hard until one night when *"it wasn't working."* He and Maxine had enjoyed sex up to that point. I asked him whether he had difficulty getting and maintaining erections during masturbation, and he said no. I asked him whether he woke up with erections, and he said he did from time to time.

"So, you used to be able to get erections with Maxine. One night you couldn't, and now that's all you worry about?" I inquired. *"And, now, you find you can get erections when you masturbate or wake up with them, but you can't get them when you're with Maxine."*

I could feel the frustration in his response, *"Yeah."*

"Ah, okay," I said. *"I imagine this has been very confusing to you. I think I understand what's happening. Here's the good news, Carl. You don't have erectile* **dysfunction**; *you have erectile* **disappointment**.*"*

As I tell so many of my patients, regardless of whether you have a penis or a vulva, you will undoubtedly experience stressful situations that feel overwhelming. Quite frankly, who hasn't? Stress can interfere with your sexual responsiveness due to the release of adrenaline and cortisol. You're in fight–or– flight mode. Concurrently, your mind goes a million miles a minute, the blinders come down, and all that you see is the problem before you. Typically, when this happens, you either respond as Carl did and withdraw into yourself or leave the room entirely, or you disregard what's happening and forge ahead with oral or manual stimulation, kissing or holding, hoping that the winds will change, bringing on a sexual response.

Here's the reality, though: sometimes, your body won't respond in ways that you demand. Your body will disappoint you on occasion. However, disappointment isn't proof that something is wrong, broken, or pathological. You might have moments where you feel psychologically and emotionally aroused, but your genitals are non-responsive. Conversely, there may be times when your genitals appear excited, but you don't have any desire. What is this all to say? Arousal Non-Concordance (i.e., the discrepancy between genital response and psychological/emotional sexual response) is normal. When it shows up, however, especially in the context of a society that demands sexual perfection, it can be pretty disappointing, embarrassing, or confusing.

In Chapter 1, I discussed the overcontrolled temperament and the high cost of having too much self-control: a sense of loneliness, interpersonal problems, over-the-top perfectionism, difficulty taking risks, and not adapting to situations. Now in Chapter 2, I'm going to illustrate how an OC temperament can be a liability in the context of sexual and intimate relationships.

Making the OC-Sexuality Connection

It bears repeating that we OCs possess many positive characteristics that have enabled us to be successful. We're the darlings of our employers and the source of envy among our colleagues because we're dutiful, hardworking, and able to delay gratification easily. We're also great at noticing details and patterns, and we aim for perfection in all that we do. Furthermore, we find comfort in following the rules and ensuring fairness; we're driven by the desire to do the right thing. These are all admirable qualities that have served us well throughout our lives.

However, those same qualities can pose problems within our sexual and intimate relationships, challenging our ability to establish and maintain long-term, romantic partnerships. For example, some OCs commit quickly to a long-term relationship to gain the safety and security of monogamy but then quickly find that their partner ceases to meet their expectations. In contrast, others delay progressing a relationship from casual to serious for fear that it would disrupt the comfort and predictability that they've established in singlehood. The latter group can also develop a complex about not having found "the one" given how successful they are in other areas of their life.

Sexually, OCs are at risk of developing problems in the bedroom (e.g., low sexual desire, erectile disappointment, inability to orgasm, premature ejaculation, painful sex, to name a few). For example, OCs pride themselves on maintaining self-control; however, the very nature of an orgasm is the total loss of control. You can imagine, then, how one's temperament can interfere with their sex life. This is the connection I want to make between your OC traits and their impact on your sexual experiences and intimacy with others.

How OC Traits Impede Sexuality

In Chapter 1, I defined the four traits of the OC temperament, using Lynch's RO DBT model, and how these traits impact the lives of many people and influence how they engage with the world. For review, these traits are (1) low receptivity and openness to the unexpected; (2) inflexible and hyper-perfectionism; (3) emotionally expressionless and unaware; and (4) undeveloped interpersonal dynamics. In the context of making nice with naughty, let's take a closer look at how these four traits can impede sexual and intimate relationships.

1. Low Receptivity and Openness to the Unexpected

Overcontrolled people are often collectors. Some collect things, which at the extreme can develop into a hoarding compulsion. Compulsive hoarding of things is fueled by the anxiety that one might need the object in the future or that someone else might need it; they don't want to be caught empty-handed. Others collect non-material items, like time (e.g., *"I need to save time; I mustn't waste time; I must be on time."*), and many collect thoughts and ideas by reading books, often self-help books, looking for the correct answers that will surely guide them through life's difficult moments. Nevertheless, regardless of what is being collected, all OC people share a compulsion to hoard safety and security, seeking solace in predictability and the familiar. Let me give you an example.

Barbara doesn't like it when her boyfriend Julius comes on to her in the middle of the week. She's a busy business owner, and each minute of her day is scheduled. Her mind tells her that she needs to *"prepare mentally for sex."* She feels anxious and hassled when Julius pursues her sexually outside the day that's been scheduled for it. Over time, Julius' libido plummets from having suppressed his desires. Sex is no longer fun for him; it's become too stressful. He sees himself as just another thing on Barbara's to-do list.

When I met with Barbara and Julius, I asked Barbara, *"I'm curious. Do you ever feel horny on other days other than Saturday night?"*

Barbara replied, *"Sometimes, but not usually."*

"What happens when you feel horny? I mean, what do you do," I asked.

She explained, *"I don't do anything. I know the moment will eventually pass. I have to focus on all of the demands on my plate. I don't have time to indulge. That's why we schedule sex for Saturdays."*

I probed cautiously, *"So, just to make sure I understand, you'll have a flash of desire and then suppress it so that you can work on your to-do list?"*

"That's right. I know that we'll have sex on Saturday."

"And when you have sex on Saturdays, do you always desire it?" I asked.

"No. It's often the case that I don't. I'm often so tired from the week. I just know that it's important for the marriage, so I do it," she replied.

I followed, *"During the times that sex is scheduled and you desire it, do you find that it makes a difference in your level of enjoyment?"*

"You bet!" she said with a smile. *"Those are special moments! I wish the stars would align like that more often."*

"I see. So, it's the rule that sex can only occur on Saturdays that prevents you from taking advantage of your experience of desire during the week, perhaps when you're less tired, even though there's a higher probability that you'd find sex more enjoyable and meaningful during these high desire moments?"

"I'm picking up what you're putting down," Barbara said with a nervous laugh.

As with so many OC people, Barbara hoarded safety and security by adhering to her schedule, attempting to treat anxieties associated with feeling vulnerable around unplanned events. When she set her mind to something, she made it happen. For example, upon meeting Julius, she knew he was the one and began planning their wedding. Once she was married, she felt like that task was achieved. She was off to the races to fulfill the next goal on her vision board. Additionally, she resisted and resented anything impeding her hyper-productivity, the source of much of her personal and professional validation. She couldn't be distracted by low-reward activities like her or her husband's sexual needs.

Vulnerability is a scary emotion among us OCs. The thought of not producing and having others think negatively of us is a source of significant anxiety. We want people to like and accept us and fear being rejected. You'll notice our discussion of the role of vulnerability throughout this book. Although a scary feeling for OCs, vulnerability is also essential in creating intimate connections. However, it takes courage to be vulnerable.

Start with an Open Heart

Whenever we think of someone with courage, we think of a bold and brave person, acting when others are afraid or simply acting without fear of failure. Courage comes from the Old French word *corage*, which derives from the Latin *cor*, meaning heart. You see, making nice with naughty all starts with the heart—an open heart—creating a chain of outcomes necessary for intimacy to flourish. An open heart is a state of being where you're open to new experiences; you accept and behave spontaneously with your partner, allowing your love and sexual expression to flow through you without obstruction. We all long to experience an open heart more often, but at times we can feel too scared and vulnerable to reveal ourselves in such a profound and exposing way.

While most couples who see me long for more intimacy, I teach them that intimacy is a product of a chain of actions preceding it, beginning with having heart-felt courage. With courage (which includes an element of fear), you can be vulnerable, experience a sequence of loving connections with your partner(s), and develop the intimacy you desire. You cannot generate more intimacy without connection, vulnerability, and courage.

Courage → Vulnerability → Connection → Intimacy

Dr. Peggy Kleinplatz's extensive interviews of everyday people having extraordinary sex lives found a common theme: many identified vulnerability and the ability to surrender to sex itself and their partner as vital elements for creating and sustaining a magnificent sex life.[3] It's difficult for OC people to be vulnerable; we're often unwilling to allow ourselves that level of defenselessness. As a result, OCs struggle with experiencing true intimacy with their partners, which some misguidedly define as closeness.

Let me explain. One of the most common complaints expressed by couples during our sessions is *"we're not close anymore."* As I dive in deeper, I find they're equating physical closeness with intimacy, but closeness and intimacy are two different things. I define closeness as low risk, low anxiety, high predictability, comfort, and familiarity. On the other hand, I define intimacy as high risk, high anxiety, low predictability, newness, and novelty, which fuel vulnerability. As mentioned before, vulnerability lies at the core of OC people's fears. I elaborate further on the differences between closeness and intimacy in Chapter 5.

---

[3] Kleinplatz, Peggy & Ménard, A (March 19, 2020). *Magnificent Sex: Lessons from Extraordinary Lovers,* pp 28–29. Routledge Publishing.
https://www.amazon.com/Magnificent-Sex-Lessons-Extraordinary-Lovers/dp/0367181371/ref=sr_1_1?crid=36QQ15Y113HZ7&keywords=Magnificent+sex&qid=1640015880&sprefix=magnificent+sex%2Caps%2C153&sr=8-1

I tell couples who bring their complaint to me about not being close that the intimacy they're seeking has to be the outcome of something. They can't flip a switch and suddenly feel intimate with each other again. The struggle is similar to trusting someone immediately after they've betrayed you. For example, after a partner is caught in an affair, the couple, hoping to salvage their marriage, embarks on a path of rebuilding trust. In the same way, intimacy comes from repeated affectionate, loving interactions, allowing yourself to be vulnerable, and trusting that your partner has your back.

Another common complaint among OCs who show low receptivity and openness is their fear of their partner changing or that their partner has changed. I'll often hear, *"They're different now; they're not like they were when we first met."*

"Of course, they've changed," I say. *"You've changed as well. But what really has changed? Is it them or your ideal of them?"*

Love infatuates us at first. It possesses us with passion and even admiration for the other person; it also blinds us to the realities of that person that are also there initially. We become way more in love with an ideal that we've formed through whatever misconceptions or misperceptions we acquired early on when dating, now propped up by our egos in defense of that model we created. Now that the couple has been together for a while, they each have sobered up, if you will, and see their partner more clearly now. So, it isn't so much that the partner has changed; instead, one is no longer misperceiving and idealizing their partner.

OCs find it challenging to live with the reality that their partner isn't as perfect as once imagined. The contrast may cause the OC partner to feel like they don't know their partner anymore. They may feel as if they got the "bait and switch." Moreover, OCs work so hard to make all aspects of their life predictable, and once it's perfectly curated, including their relationships, they work just as hard to avoid disruptions.

Consequently, OCs' low threshold for the unexpected compels them to categorize people and put them into boxes that are definable, predictable, and non-threatening. OCs find it very hard to accept that their partner has changed and that they're living with someone who's still an unfolding mystery.

"Of course, they've changed. You've changed, too, and your perception of them has also changed," I advise. *"Your need for intimacy requires vulnerability, and vulnerability requires letting go of that ideal."*

Suppose you've identified that intimacy is missing in your relationship. In that case, there's a high probability that there's been a breakdown somewhere earlier in that chain described above. Under closer scrutiny, you may find that you struggle with connecting to things of interest, being comfortable feeling vulnerable, or having the courage and the heart to put yourself in context and recognize the need to turn down the overcontrolledness in your life. A fulfilling intimate and sexual relationship requires higher receptivity and adaptability to change and an openness to the unexpected.

2. Inflexible and Hyper-Perfectionist

This second OC trait centers on rules and perfectionism. Think about it. You're great at noticing when things aren't right, like that picture across the room that's just slightly crooked, the social faux pas you made at dinner, or the grammatical errors in this book. Things that aren't right stick out to you like a proverbial sore thumb. You have an aptitude for organizing information, seeing patterns, and identifying what has to happen to make things right. Over the years, you've acquired and refined a list of rules to live by and believe that others would be best served by living by those rules as well.

As an OC myself, I've established a terrible habit of hyper-focusing on people's language—both spoken and unspoken, which is a superpower for a psychotherapist! Tangentially, the difference between a friend and a therapist is that a friend listens to what you say, but a therapist also listens to what you don't say. However, the liability is that my OC-brain also goes into hyper-alert when people misuse words (e.g., *irregardless* instead of *regardless*). When I was a teen, I developed the terrible habit of correcting others' grammar to the point where my older sister took me aside and told me that it wasn't polite and that people don't want to be friends with people who make them feel under the microscope. She was so right!

Nevertheless, bad habits die hard. While I've indeed turned down my "critique of language" in everyday conversations, my inner sentinel stands at attention during arguments. To my chagrin, I laser focus on what's being said. *Are their words precise? Are they stating their position correctly? Are we fighting about the same thing?* Unfortunately, this defense mechanism leaves the other unnerved. They've come to me as a partner with concerns, and now there's a fight about something else; ultimately, they don't feel particularly heard. (I've worked to turn the volume down on this defense mechanism using strategies identified later in this book.)

Perhaps you find yourself rigidly attached to your expectations, preferences, and rules. Frank, a corporate executive, and Elizabeth, an accountant, have been married for 18 years. Frank and Elizabeth found a strong connection around their interest in healthy living. They both grew up as athletes and took pride in their appearance. However, over 18 years, Frank has *"just let himself go,"* according to Elizabeth, who continues to faithfully exercise daily.

"He's got a beer belly now," she continued. *"I just don't find him sexually attractive. I mean, I've told him so many times over the years that I want him to get to the weight when we were in high school. He looked great then. He didn't have that belly."*

Frank acknowledges that he's gained weight. He attributes it to being in a job where business meals are common, combined with sitting at his desk all day. While he exercises regularly, he doesn't burn off enough calories to compensate for his caloric intake. But there's something more going on here. Frank's not confident that even the weight loss will reduce his partner's criticisms lodged against him. *"Elizabeth seems to nitpick everything,"* as Frank puts it, *"not just with me but with the kids, too. The general message is that none of us are good enough, and we're just a pain in her ass."*

Elizabeth suffers from a common problem among OCs known as *sexual perfectionism* (SP), which is an expectation that one's sexual expressions are perfect.[4] There are generally four dimensions of SP: (1) the expectations and perfectionistic standards that you place on yourself as a sexual partner, (2) the expectations and standards that you place on others as sexual partners, (3) the perception that your partner demands you be sexually perfect, and (4) the perception that society expects you to meet sexual standards perfectly. For Elizabeth, her perfectionist standard is that her partner Frank must not have a beer belly for her to be sexually attracted to him. Other SP standards could include beliefs such as:

- I *must* get an erection for sex to be meaningful.
- My partner *must* get an erection, or else I question my self-worth and attractiveness.
- I *must* bring my partner to orgasm. My partner must bring me to orgasm.
- My partner *must* desire me sexually for me to feel attractive.
- My partner expects me to be perfect or expects parts of my body to be perfect.
- If there is emotional distance between us, even if I'm horny, I mustn't pursue my partner sexually until he apologizes first.

---

[4] Stoeber, J., Harvey, L.N. *Multidimensional Sexual Perfectionism and Female Sexual Function: A Longitudinal Investigation. Archives of Sexual Behavior* 45, 2003–2014 (2016). https://doi.org/10.1007/s10508-016-0721-7

- My partner and I *must* have an orgasm for sex to be legitimate.

Sexual perfectionism is also known to interfere with an essential phase of the sexual response cycle, namely the *excitement stage*, when your body is ramping up for sexual activity. Kurt, an engineer, and Hillary, a lawyer, have been married for 11 years. They report having a great friendship, which has remained solid despite the many stressors of careers and parenthood. What their life is completely lacking is any sexual relationship. They have not had sex in several years though the problems began years earlier.

After meeting with the couple, I realized that Kurt was OC and had SP. He lacked sexual confidence and worried whether he was *"doing it right."* Sure, when they wanted to get pregnant, it was off to the races; there was a job to do, and the OC in Kurt was going to make sure it got done. But, as soon as Hillary became pregnant, the couple returned to their sexless routine of being friends.

In short, sexual perfectionism can suppress the excitement stage. Kurt's performance concerns decreased his sexual self-esteem while increasing his anxiety and displeasure in having sex with Hillary. Additionally, when one feels that their partner is a hyper-perfectionist, they'll likely experience arousal issues such as erectile disappointment or difficulty with lubrication.

What are your rules about sex? What are your *musts, shoulds,* and *have tos?* In the space below, list out the rules that your mind says must be satisfied to enjoy sex. If you can't identify any rules, ask your partner what they've observed; they might have some helpful insights.

Rules that Must Be Satisfied:

3. Emotionally Expressionless and Unaware

A common characteristic of this third OC trait in the context of sexual and intimate relationships is that OCs spend considerable time in their heads, overthinking things to the point of denying their physical needs and desires. We can come across as emotionally disengaged, poker-faced, and absent any signs of interest or engagement. For example, if we're thrilled, anxious, or depressed, there's a high probability that no one would know it. Instead, we hide the pain or discontent behind a façade that suggests to others that everything is under control.

While hiding one's emotions may be innate for OCs, many of us also grew up in families where emotional suppression was expected. For example, I learned early that I had to demonstrate sufficient appreciation to my mother if she gave me a gift. If I didn't express adequate excitement, she would become upset with me. So, I learned to pretend I was excited out of consideration for my mom and her expectations of me.

It's similar to when a woman fakes an orgasm. She would rather deny the reality that she's not receiving sufficient stimulation and deny herself expressing her uneasiness with sex than risk making her partner uncomfortable or the moment awkward. The fake orgasm becomes her illusion of sexual enjoyment for herself and her partner to protect her feelings of vulnerability.

In addition to being emotionally expressionless, OC people can be physically disengaged, in a sense denying themselves any feeling of physical enjoyment. In Chapter 1, I gave an example of this when I explained how rules-driven OC women, when horny, will not pursue their sexual pleasure or let their partner pursue them if it means inadvertently reinforcing their partner's "bad behavior."

Being emotionally and physically expressionless also means that OC people consistently under-report their sex-related distresses. For example, it's less common for women to talk about vaginal sex being painful. It's never been a socially acceptable topic of conversation. On the other hand, it's normal to talk about how uncomfortable anal sex can be because it's expected that it might be painful. Rather than acknowledging and reporting their sexual pain to their partner, OC women will turn down sex instead of risk feeling vulnerable by talking about their experiences. Moreover, OC women experience pressures to reinforce social expectations that sex is always enjoyable. Unfortunately, their male partners are often unaware of their distress and assume they're doing something wrong when their female partner expresses pain.

Conversely, other OC men and women might exclusively pursue medical explanations for their sexual problems rather than face the possibility that their sexual issues are a product of emotional, psychological, and relational distress. In short, it's less vulnerable to seek medical advice in search of biological causes for erectile issues, painful sex, and problems with orgasms and libido than to have difficult conversations with their partner about emotional and relationship needs. Unfortunately, this approach often leads to frustration and more hopelessness when no medical reasons are found that explain their sexual issues. At this time, medical providers are likely to recommend seeing a sex therapist.

4. Undeveloped Interpersonal Dynamics

This fourth trait that an OC portrays is low social connectedness and an emotional detachment from others. Many will struggle with bonding emotionally or attaching to others and are often uncomfortable connecting physically. Physical touch, a staple of intimacy and healthy familial relationships, can be a point of contention for many OCs and their partners. OCs manage anxiety over holding hands, hugging, and kissing by establishing and enforcing rules discouraging public displays of affection, which only reinforces the perception that OCs are cold and aloof.

"We just weren't a hugging family."

Jordan and his husband, Lewis, came to see me for couple's therapy. Lewis shared that he felt increasingly neglected by Jordan's lack of emotional and physical reciprocity and worried Jordan wouldn't answer his pleas for change.

Partway through the session, I asked Jordan, *"What was it like for you growing up in a family where you weren't hugged?"*

"I don't know…it was okay, I guess."

"Just okay? That sounds like an understatement. Did it feel like something was missing?

"Yeah, I suppose so. I was envious of my friends whose families showed physical and verbal affection. I mean, I don't remember being hugged much, and it wasn't until I was in high school before hearing my dad tell me he loved me."

"Ouch! I'm sorry to hear that. So, you were missing both physical and verbal affection? I wonder whether you felt like you just didn't belong, that you were in some ways an outsider."

"I still do. But, that's okay; it happens."

"And so now you find yourself in a situation where there is little physical or verbal affection?"

Jordan reflected, *"Yeah. Seems so. I mean, it just wasn't something that was taught in my family."*

"I get it," I said. *"It seems like that's a tradition and legacy you honor and want to be repeated in your marriage with Lewis?"*

"I don't think so. It really isn't."

"Well, is there evidence you want to **dishonor** *that legacy by demonstrating physical and verbal affection in this relationship? I mean, based on what I heard, the evidence suggests that you're still trying to be the 'good son' and keep the legacy of 'not being a hugging family' alive,"* I said tongue-in-cheek.

Jordan chuckled, then said pensively, *"I never thought of it that way. But you're right. The evidence does suggest that. I mean, when I think about it, I've always been afraid someone would get too close to me and end up not liking what they see. When you see other kids' parents act affectionately, but your parents don't, you wonder whether it's about you. I definitely see a pattern of keeping people at arm's length. They can't hurt me from 'over there.'"*

As with so many of us OCs, Jordan is an internal processor. OCs can quickly get stuck in mental loops of mind-chatter that interfere with our relationships with people and things outside ourselves. I bet that if you're like Jordan, anxious or depressed, no one would ever know (except very close family and friends). You've learned how to maintain a poker face, show little expression, and create the illusion that everything is under control. I bet that when people ask how you're doing, one of your standard replies is *"I'm fine,"* even when you aren't fine.

The reality, of course, is that we're social creatures whose optimal living is dependent on an interdependent web of relationships. Those close to you need to trust that you have their back, which you're remarkably good at doing. You (yes, *you*!) also need to know that others have your back as well.

Of course, there will be times when others will misuse your acts of vulnerability, and you'll get hurt. Yet, I suspect, if you look over the course of your life, you've survived many incidences of hurt. So, it isn't like being hurt is new to you. I also suspect you've experienced a lot of pain over the years that have been left unspoken for fear of burdening someone or fear others would see your pain as inconsequential. The temptation is to use these moments of hurt as reasons to avoid opening your heart and risking vulnerability again. However, the tax you pay is to continue to feel isolated and alone.

These four traits that I've just shared with you define the OC temperament and how we OCs engage with the world. Yet while they personify the necessary qualities that have served us well throughout our lives, they are also the reason for the stress and dissatisfaction you're experiencing in your sexual life and the challenges you have in your ability to establish and maintain long-term romantic relationships.

My Goal Is Not to Make You Undercontrolled

I want to emphasize, though, that I have no desire for OC people to become under-controlled. My goal isn't to make an OC, like you and me, an under-controlled person. I often tell my patients that there aren't enough drugs or therapy in the world that will make me under-controlled. That's not my goal, and it doesn't have to be your goal either. Not that there's anything wrong with being under-controlled. I love under-controlled people. They're spontaneous and light-hearted. I admire how they can step on the dance floor without a sip of alcohol to have a good time. Still, while I like who I am, I've recognized that there are times when being a little less OC would be good for me.

Ultimately, *Making Nice with Naughty* is designed to help you turn down the volume on the OC so you can have more of what you need and desire for yourself and your partner. That's most likely what led you to pick up my book in the first place, so let's dive into this together. In the next chapter, we'll begin with a closer examination of your inner voice, which I call the ego. The ego is the narrator of your life, prodding you to buy thoughts, many of which aren't true, and preventing you from having a quieted mind.

CHAPTER 3
LET GO OF MY EGO

Do I contradict myself?
Very well then, I contradict myself,
(I am large, I contain multitudes.)

— **Walt Whitman**

You may recall Kellogg's "Let go of my Eggo" TV commercial that aired in the 1970s. It depicted a brother having a tug-of-war with his sister, who refuses to let go of his breakfast waffle. In the context of making nice with naughty, your tug-of-war isn't with a sister stealing your breakfast, but instead the conflict is with your inner voice—the narrator of your life—which I refer to as the ego. I draw on the Buddhist psychology's notion of ego, not the Freudian notion, in helping you understand your experience as an OC person wanting more out of your sex and intimate relationships. The Buddhists identified that inner voice as representing your conditioned self, a self that has been curated over time by external influences (e.g., parents, school, culture, religious institutions, etc.). You may find yourself wrestling with your ego around sex and sexuality, thus preventing you from expressing and finding enjoyment in your sexuality and maintaining long-term intimate relationships.

Essentially, the ego is the you that you tell yourself you are. It's your mind chatter, which constantly compares things: good/bad, right/wrong, just/unjust, fair/unfair. Moreover, your overcontrolled ego regularly compares you to your ideal self, the coworker whose desk you pass each day, or some perceived standard set by your family, spiritual community, or social group. The ego thus is the embodiment of your inner critic and that which prevents you from having a quieted mind.

A common complaint among OC people is that they can never silence their mind chatter, especially during lovemaking. Instead, their thoughts race at a million miles a minute, leaving them stressed and worn out. Just look at your own experience and how your distracting, interrupting, highly-opinionated inner voice makes it nearly impossible to experience an enjoyable sex life. I'll illustrate that challenge throughout this chapter.

However, it's helpful to understand that the ego isn't the enemy here. The ego is motivated to help you navigate the world and avoid anticipated pain and discomfort, which it does by focusing on past or future. The ego assumes that ruminating on past or future events will help solve problems and thereby avoid suffering. However, when the ego over-focuses on the past, you'll likely experience various feelings of depression. When the ego over-focuses on the future, you'll experience various forms of anxiety. While some OCs can focus on the past and the rules and expectations that command our thoughts and actions, most find that their egos focus near exclusively on the future and what could possibly go wrong. Sound familiar? The ego believes it can plan for and mitigate anticipated problems by concentrating on and planning for the future. Let me give you a typical example.

Chip and Kerrie have traveled the world. They've visited many countries in Europe as well as traveled throughout Asia, South America, and a few countries in Africa. Though they love to travel, Chip spends many hours planning the itinerary. He stresses about the tiniest of details, wanting the vacation to be perfect but, more precisely, wanting to ensure that nothing bad happens. Even his contingency plans have contingency plans. Kerrie enjoys the travel but admits that Chip's stress leading up to the vacation stresses her out, too. She feels compelled to go along with Chip's plans because he worked so hard to iron them out. However, Kerrie has found that the itineraries leave little room for impromptu experiences, to explore off the beaten path, and enjoy unexpected delights.

However, the ego doesn't always ruminate on the future, like Chip's ego. Sometimes it can stress over the (unknown) future and then transition to a focus on the past, creating the perfect conditions for depression. I'll give you a personal example. Years ago, I intended to write my first book over the summer. In January of that year, I routinely fantasized about writing that manuscript and the sense of accomplishment I would feel in completing it. As spring passed, I made very little progress in organizing and preparing my ideas and material for the book. Everything around me was blooming but me. As summer rolled on, I still hadn't progressed, and by the end of the season, I realized that I had accomplished nothing and grew increasingly depressed when I reflected on the time that passed. That fall marked the most profound depression that I had ever experienced. I felt ashamed that I hadn't met my expectation.

Many OCs are decisive in developing and establishing goals, making consistent progress toward those goals, and crossing the finish line strong. The ego admonishes you to delay gratification for a more successful and worthy outcome, usually by repeated statements of "*I must...,*" "*I should...,*" "*I have to....*". Such egos are way more interested in the *wanting* of something in the future (i.e., the outcome of a goal met) than being interested in *having* what's available now (e.g., a pleasurable sexual experience).

However, not all OCs are born alike. Some are burdened with an ego that has its own agendas and focuses on criticizing or finding fault in the past or present. One such agenda is fear of having disappointed someone and not measuring up. Indeed, this is the case among OCs whose egos are obsessed with sexual perfectionism, constantly wrestling with themselves by asking, *"Am I doing this right?" "Is my body sexy enough in the way they want me to be?" "Am I competent?" "Am I good enough?"*

In Chapter 2, Carl's inner critic berated him for not getting an erection that one time. Now his ego is convincing him to pull away from Maxine and eliminate the possibility of repeating that embarrassment. His ego is afraid that being physically close and intimate with her will escalate into something sexual, and he will fail again. Consequently, his worrying triggers Maxine's anxiety. It makes her question her attractiveness and causes her to resent Carl for not being open with her, all of which is taken a heavy toll on their relationship.

The overcontrolled temperament becomes increasingly maladaptive when the inner voice constantly compares and self-criticizes. Consequently, the OC can't effectively adjust to the environment or situation in which they find themselves—their mind is too distracted. In time, the inner critic can convince you that you're not good enough or that you'll never measure up. Sometimes, that inner critic is turned outward and questions whether your partner is good enough and perhaps you chose wrong, which drives a wedge further between you.

OCs struggle with insecurity. While the world "out there" would never know that the OC person questions their competence, capabilities, or effectiveness, the OC knows their own mind chatter. When OCs face situations that trigger insecurity, their ego adopts a mindset to manage the anxiety associated with the situation. Thomas Lynch, Ph.D., whom you met in Chapter 1, calls these the Fixed and Fatalistic Mindsets.[5]

---

[5] Lynch (n 1), pp 8–21.

A Fixed Mindset

Recall Barbara from Chapter 2 who didn't appreciate her husband Julius coming on to her in the middle of her busy week. I used her and Julius' story to illustrate one of the four traits of an OC person: low receptivity and openness to the unexpected. Over time, Julius' desire for Barbara diminished, and sex stopped being fun and fulfilling. Instead, it became a scheduled weekend routine, like cleaning the house or mowing the lawn.

A fixed mindset has its sights laser-focused on achieving a specific outcome. It's a form of psychological rigidity often expressed as moralism, certainty, and self-righteousness. It's an unchanging attitude, independent and unmindful of any new information notifying us that the situation has now changed. Of course we all need to make room in our thinking and beliefs and adapt to changing conditions, but those considerations would diminish the ego, which is why OCs tend to ignore feedback.

"I have this goal, and I'm not going to change" is what the fixed mindset of an OC thinks to itself, bolstered by all kinds of self-convincing moralities. *"Whatever happens, I'm going to forge right through. I must get to my goal."* OCs have an unwavering conviction, reinforced by the belief that they already have the answers. In Barbara's case, her ego's fixed rule is that sex between her and her partner can only happen on Saturdays even if she's horny on a Wednesday or Julius is interested. There is no time to indulge; Barbara is psychologically compelled to stick to her plan and routine and mustn't waver from the productivity of the workweek.

We can see the effect Barbara's fixed thinking has on Julius; desire and passion do not like too much premeditation. In my work with couples, once each person has separately identified their sexual ritual (i.e., their process for engaging in sex, such as who touches whom first; who kisses whom first; what genitals are touched first), I'll have the couple merge their narratives to see if one story surfaces. If there's a high degree of agreement, there's likely a great deal of rigidity in their sexual ritual. If you know that every time you have sex, it will happen the same way, it diminishes your motivation to have it again. The act of sex becomes static and desireless and loses any sense of vitality.

A Fatalistic Mindset

Not all OCs have fixed mindsets. Some respond to unexpected events in a more dramatic fashion. They become fatalistic, fearing that what will happen in the future cannot be changed, and resign themselves to the worst possibility. Carl's reaction to not getting an erection is typical of the fatalistic mindset. Feeling powerless and hopeless, he resigns to a sexless relationship with Maxine. *"I'm not going to have sex at all. I embarrass myself every damn time. I'm just a failure at it. I'm just going to go to work each day, come home each evening, hide in my man cave, and play video games. I don't need more of a relationship."*

When one doesn't get what one wants, the fatalistic mindset interferes with sexual expression and fulfillment because it results in giving up, over-accommodating, pacifying, and withdrawing into oneself. Carl expects an erection on demand as if dicks are dildos. When he realizes nothing will get his dick up—not what he's imagining doing to Maxine or what Maxine is doing to him—he throws his hands up in defeat instead.

The fatalistic mindset often includes feelings of anxiety and awkwardness, even fear of pursuing sex. OCs with this outlook might retreat from sexual activity altogether. By allowing his inner critic to run his life, Carl ignores the feedback that his partner is unhappy sexually. Their relationship is crumbling, yet his inner critic will not allow him to confront his anxieties and fears so that he and Maxine can realize their sexual potential.

You Are Not Your Mind Chatter

Here's a little secret: that voice you hear in your head—that narrator of your life—isn't *you*! YOU are who notices the voice. *You* are the awareness behind the voice. I know, it sounds woo-woo, right? Maybe even a bit too radical? I get it but think about it. For nearly your whole life, you may have judged yourself for specific thoughts you had, as if those thoughts were a reflection of your entire personhood. Well, I'm here to tell you that it wasn't you that was doing the judging; it was your ego's overcontrolled nature.

If there's any hope of turning down your OC dial, you need to start embracing the real *you* from a higher perspective. What I mean to say is that *you* are not your experience; *you* are who observes your experience. For example, you may have routinely said to yourself, *"I'm anxious."* However, under closer scrutiny, *you* aren't anxious; instead, *you* are the awareness of the feeling of anxiety inside of you. There's *you*, and then there is the experience you are observing. You can't be both *you* AND the experience. This makes me recall a conversation with a patient not that long ago and her experience of coming to understand the meaning of a higher perspective and creating a space between her and her experiences.

> *"What do you mean my anxiety can't hurt me; it certainly seems like it's hurting me,"* Tory blurted.
>
> *"I know, Tory,"* I began, *"it sounds confusing because your experience suggests something else."*
>
> *"Definitely."*
>
> *"Well, would you be willing to allow me to share a metaphor that I think might help?"* I offered.
>
> *"Sure,"* Tory replied, somewhat skeptical of what would come.
>
> *"Great. Take a look out the window. See those clouds? Your thoughts and feelings are like those clouds. They appear quite real and even solid. Yet, we know that they're not solid masses. You've flown through clouds, right?"* I asked, to which she nodded.

I went on, *"And isn't it the case that those clouds can come together and even bring dark skies, which might lead to thunderstorms, tornadoes, or even powerful hurricanes?"*

Tory nodded again.

"And yet, no matter how dark and scary the sky gets or how violent those clouds act on one another, does any of it damage the sky?"

"Are you saying that I'm the sky," asked Tory.

"You're here, aren't you? Isn't the evidence that you've survived every cloud, dark sky, and violent thunderstorm that's ever happened to you?"

Tory thought for a moment. *"I suppose so, but it can be tough to see that at times. It all feels like it's right in front of me."*

"Let's try another experiment then," I suggested. *"Take your hands and bring them together like a prayer. Now, open them as if they were pages of a book. Now bring the book up to your face with only a quarter of an inch of space between your face and hands. Can you see me?"*

"No."

"Good. These pages blocking your view are all of the thoughts of the ego. When you believe that your mind-chatter is who you are, the ego blocks your ability to see beyond the thoughts and judgments of your mind. It's the only thing you see and experience; thus, you're led to believe that you are your experience. Yet I still exist beyond your hands. I'm still here. I see all of you despite you only seeing your hands."

It was as if a veil fell from Tory's eyes. *"I get it now. I need to create more space between me and my experience."*

"Well, imagine that! What would it be like to feel less tethered to the stories that your mind is telling you?" I asked.

"Oh my God, it would be so much less stressful. I could finally relax," Tory exclaimed.

Does That Thought Feel Heavy or Light?

Tory isn't alone. Most people walk this earth feeling that they and their mind chatter are the same, and the consequences of the conclusion that they're drawing are evident. Now don't get me wrong, the ego isn't inherently bad. However, the unregulated ego can lead to emotional, mental, and relationship problems facing so many OCs. The good news is that we can begin to regulate our egos by questioning the thoughts that they produce. We don't have to examine every thought; we only have to question the stressful ones.

Listen to your mind chatter and evaluate whether the thought running through your head feels light or heavy. Generally speaking, heavy thoughts correlate with feeling stressed. When you have a stressful and heavy thought, that's a clue that you bought into a thought that isn't true. Why? I can say this with certitude because, without exception, the truth always feels light, not heavy and stressful. Now, it's important to point out that the lightness of the truth isn't synonymous with the truth being pain-free. Sometimes the truth is excruciatingly painful, although painful and heavy aren't synonymous either. Let me explain.

Someone's child goes missing, and for months there's no news, no break in the case. Imagine the pain and anguish the parents are experiencing, not knowing whether their child is alive or dead. Nine months go by before they hear a knock at the door from a state trooper. When their eyes greet each other, the trooper informs them: *"Mr. and Ms. Smith, we regret to say that we believe we found your daughter's body. We'll need you to come with us to confirm."*

There seems to be a general pattern in agonizing scenarios as we process through pain, anguish, and relief. The relief comes from the parents no longer enduring the heaviness of pain and worrying. They say, *"It's a relief just to know the truth."* The truth lifted the burden of not knowing. That's not to say that the truth feels good, but the truth solves the mystery and lightens their burden.

Winning the Tug-of-War

The ego churns out thoughts; that's its job. However, not all thoughts are problems. When you're planning something—say, journaling or listening to a podcast—you're generating thoughts and using your mind as a tool. However, when you're stressed, that's the evidence that your ego uses your mind to buy into thoughts that aren't true—your mind is using you as a tool. Many people fail to observe their thinking from a sky-level view and don't realize that their ego is winning the internal tug-of-war.

Byron Katie is the originator of a simple yet powerful process for letting go of the ego. Katie's process, called *The Work*, is a method of inquiry designed to ask and listen for answers one finds inside and to open their mind to potentially life-transforming insights.[6] The method is about questioning mind chatter and creating more space between you and your experiences.

There are two phases in Katie's method: (1) isolating one of your thoughts and inspecting that thought by asking four specific questions and (2) turning your thoughts about it around to see if the opposite is true or truer than your original beliefs. Katie proposes that you begin the process by asking these four questions about a specific belief that your inner voice has imposed on you:

1. Is [the thought] true? (Yes or no. If no, move to question 3.)
2. Can you absolutely know that it's true? (Yes or no)

---

[6] Katie, Byron (December 7, 2021). *Loving What Is: Four Questions That Can Change Your Life*, pp 17–21. Harmony Books. Retrieved from https://www.amazon.com/Loving-What-Revised-Questions-Change/dp/0593234510/ref=sr_1_1?crid=26U7G57QBSKPW&dchild=1&keywords=loving+what+is+revised+edition&qid=1634653945&sprefix=loving+what+is+revised+%2Caps%2C250&sr=8-1&asin=0593234510&revisionId=&format=4&depth=1

3. How do you react? What happens when you believe that thought?
4. Whom or what would you be without the thought?

Let's apply Katie's methodology to our discussion of sexual intimacy and relationships. Carl's stressful thought is that Maxine will think he's sexually inept because he can't keep an erection. To the first question, Carl asks himself, *"Is it true that Maxine will think that I'm sexually inept because I can't keep my erection?"* to which Carl answers, *"Yes."*

He then moves on to the second question. *"Can I absolutely know that Maxine will think I'm sexually inept because I can't keep the erection?"* Carl concedes that he can't **absolutely** know that it's true that Maxine will think negatively of him.

Moving onto question #3, Carl responds, *"I start to get anxious and withdraw into myself when I imagine Maxine thinking negatively of me. I'm stressed whenever she touches me out of fear that she'll want to have sex and I won't be able to perform. It makes me want to spend less time with her."*

Finally, Carl addresses the fourth question: *Whom or what would I be without the thought that Maxine will think I'm sexually inept?"* He answers without hesitation. *"I'd be less stressed. I'd be more engaged with Maxine. I'd also be less concerned about my penis and more interested in just enjoying my time with her if I was free from that thought."*

Here's the thing: Katie's exercise isn't about *not* having the thought. It's not possible to force thoughts out of your mind and keep them out; it's just not how the mind works. Try it if you don't believe me—try not to think of a banana. What happened? Right, you thought of a banana. That's how the mind works. The mind is additive; it's not subtractive. The mind doesn't work on the same principles that exist in the world outside of the mind. For example, when you're done with this book, and it no longer serves a valuable purpose for you, you could just throw it away. (I will haunt you to the end of my days if you do!)

However, you can't rid yourself of a thought. You have to engage the thought with inquiry to change your relationship with it. *The Work* provides a simple method for challenging your ego to free yourself of heavy beliefs that have robbed you of sexual and relationship satisfaction.

Questioning his mind chatter helped Carl see that his belief that Maxine would judge him was at the core of his issue. Without the belief that she would judge him, he'd feel less stressed. In other words, his belief that Maxine would judge him caused him considerable distress. The insights from this method of inquiry don't just stop there. Katie proposes an additional step where Carl is invited to deepen the questioning process by posing "turnarounds," statements that reflect the variations of the opposites of the stressful thought. The goal is to see if one or more turnarounds are just as true or even truer than the initial stressful thought. A stressful thought can have up to three turnarounds:

> **Stressful thought**: *"Maxine will think I'm sexually inept because I can't keep an erection."*
>
> Turnaround 1: *"Maxine WON'T think that I'm sexually inept because I can't keep an erection."*
>
> Turnaround 2: *"I will think Maxine is sexually inept because I can't keep an erection."*
>
> Turnaround 3: *"I will think I'm sexually inept because I can't keep an erection."*

Carl instantly realizes that the last statement is the truest of them all. In short, he begins to understand that he's projecting his insecurity onto Maxine. Moreover, Carl acknowledges that the first statement is worth further inquiry. Namely, he can find plenty of evidence where Maxine is supportive and encouraging. If Maxine has become upset, it's likely because he's withdrawn so much over the past several weeks.

Through additional conversations with me, Carl understands that he has little control over what Maxine thinks or how she feels. And when he focuses too much on her inner experience with him, it fills him with anxiety and impacts how he relates to her.

Byron Katie offers additional gems to help Carl create space between himself and his ego. Katie encourages anyone experiencing stressful thoughts to ask themselves, *"Whose business am I in at this moment?"* She reminds her readers that there are three types of business: (1) your business, (2) NOT your business but their business, and (3) God's/universe's business (i.e., what you and no one else has control over).[7]

Let's see what happens when Carl and I apply Katie's question to his sexual difficulty. *"Carl, whose business are you in when you're worried about how Maxine will think or feel?"* I ask.

"I'm in Maxine's business," Carl answers.

"And when you're minding Maxine's business, who's minding yours?" I inquire.

Carl replies, *"No one, I suppose."*

"And, then who suffers?" I ask.

"Me."

"Right."

As illustrated through my work with Carl in helping him frame his inquiry process, freedom begins to emerge when you question your mind chatter. By calling out and probing your stressful thoughts, they lose their power over you. I believe that this method of inquiry can help set you free from what your OC ego has convinced you to be true.

---

[7] The Work of Byron Katie. *Whose Business Are You In?* At Home with BK on Zoom. Retrieved from https://thework.com/2006/09/whose-business-are-you-minding/

More, the method helps you to let go of the ego by providing a framework for embracing the real *you* from a higher perspective. From here, you can create a mindful space between you and your experiences.

Byron Katie offers free downloadable worksheets at www.thework.com that will guide you, step by step, through the method. At the end of this chapter, I've also provided a workspace where you can apply Byron Katie's inquiry process specifically to the tug-of-war you may be having in your intimate relationship with your partner.

It's Not That Complicated

Dr. Albert Ellis is another important figure from whom I draw insights that will help you in your journey in making nice with naughty. Ellis is regarded by many as the grandfather of cognitive-behavioral therapy. His innovative straight-talk approach to psychotherapy made him one of the most provocative yet influential figures in modern Western psychology. Dr. Ellis developed his approach to psychotherapy, Rational Emotive Behavior Therapy (REBT), in the 1950s to challenge the slow-moving methodology of Freudian psychoanalysis. Psychoanalysis was the dominant psychotherapeutic treatment at the time, which maintained that an exhaustive exploration of one's childhood experience was critical to understanding neurosis and curing it.[8] Ellis disagreed.

The premise of Dr. Ellis's work was that human suffering wasn't that complicated, and he believed in short-term therapy that called on his patients to focus on what was happening in their lives at that very moment and take immediate action to change their behavior. He bolstered his technique by integrating teachings from the ancient philosophies, namely Stoicism and Epicureanism, in pursuit of enduring happiness.

---

[8] The Albert Ellis Institute. *About Albert Ellis, Ph.D*. Retrieved from https://albertellis.org/about-albert-ellis-phd/.

Though I'll be covering REBT in greater detail in Chapter 7, I mention it now because Dr. Ellis's experience in helping patients realize the root cause of their suffering is what I observe with my patients today—that the primary cause of their unhappiness is rarely the situation, but their thoughts about the situation. As I shared earlier, our ego prevents us from having a quiet mind. If left unchallenged and unquestioned, the ego will strengthen in its capacity to narrate our lives and create distress and unfulfillment in our sexual and intimate relationships.

Feeding the Dragon

Sharon wants to role-play during sex, but Jim doesn't; he says it makes him feel awkward and vulnerable. A large part of my session with Jim was to help him realize that every time he doesn't do something because he's anxious or afraid, he feeds the dragon, a metaphor I use to describe the fire-breather that represents all of our egoic-based anxieties and fears.

When couples come in to see me, their dragon is obese from constant feeding. Worse yet, instead of taking measures to slay the monster, they run around the village waving their arms and yelling, *"There's a dragon in the cave! There's a dragon in the cave! Isn't it so terrible?!? What are we going to do?"*

Instead of feeding his dragon, Jim can slay the beast by facing his fear of awkwardness and vulnerability. Unfortunately, OC people are often hoarders of safety and security, fueled by fears of vulnerability where they'll be exposed and feel insecure. Jim's ego tells him that feeling awkward is intolerable and thus something must be wrong with role-playing between sex partners if it feels uncomfortable. Consequently, Jim's inner critic also tells him to immediately shut down Sharon's role-playing request, which only serves to feed his dragon and leaves Sharon feeling dismissed and undesired.

With continued avoidance, the dragon gets bigger as Jim continues to follow his ego's rules. Should this pattern persist, he risks waking up one day to realize that he hadn't had sex with his wife in years. Suppose Jim was willing to bring his anxiety and awkwardness to the cave. In that case, he could stare down his dragon, withhold its nourishment, conceive of turnarounds that are just as true or truer than what his monster is leading him to believe, and starve his fears out of existence.

The Flexible Mindset

Earlier I shared how the fixed and fatalistic mindsets are the two most prevalent defenses of our ego. Well, there's another: the flexible mindset, an attitude that OCs can adopt to improve their sexual and intimate relationships. The parallel to an adaptable mind is the sky metaphor used earlier, where you are the sky and not the clouds and storms formed by your mind chatter. You're bigger than these distractions. You are the sky, so powerful that it can contain all. By letting go of your ego, accepting the situation for what it is, and making adjustments accordingly, you acquire greater flexibility and adaptability. A flexible mindset includes a willingness to modify your goals and relax expectations for a greater emphasis on the here and now. When you think about it, the flexible mindset is the transition from the performance-based sex common among OC people to pleasure-based sex, the realization of greater openness to spontaneity and the unexpected.

My suggestion to Carl and Maxine is that there will be times when Carl will want to have an erection, but one doesn't stand at attention. I tell him that he can feed that dragon by catastrophizing, or he can reduce his reliance on his erection and use other means of helping Maxine experience pleasure. I tell him that if he were to wear a strap-on dildo, he's guaranteed to have an erection. It may not be his erection, but it's an erection, and it can then be used to have an intimate pleasure-based experience with Maxine. With a flexible mindset, there's no rule that says sex is only legitimate if it's with an erection.

The other thing I suggested to Carl is that, when experiencing erectile disappointment in the future, adapt to the situation. As he sat there next to Maxine, I said, *"Straighten and stiffen your index and middle fingers together and make them as rigid as possible so as not to lose that stiffness."* I then asked Maxine, *"Now, grab those two fingers and try to bend them,"* and she couldn't. Neither could she hide the glimmer in her eye that this little exercise created.

No matter how anxious or awkward Carl may feel, he always has two rigid fingers for his partner. Anxiety and adrenaline, regardless of how high they may be, cannot diminish erect fingers. When you are pleasure-focused, by focusing on your partner and pursuing pleasure, you use what's available to have a good time. Your partner will reciprocate by communicating their experience of pleasure, which is sensually pleasing and a turn-on for many. Not surprisingly, holders of a flexible mindset will likely find their bodies responding to the sexual stimuli now that the pressure to perform a specific way has been lessened.

It's important to point out that this process and mental orientation isn't limited to men only. Patients experiencing vaginal dryness, for example, which occurs for a range of reasons—from hormonal changes or medication side effects to emotional and psychological issues, such as a lack of desire or even anxiety—can find ways to pleasure their partner by some other means. Partners will reciprocate by communicating their experience of pleasure, which many find sensually pleasing and a turn-on. Not surprisingly, the floodgates tend to open up with the pressure off and anxiety of not getting wet a distant thought.

Gag Your Inner Critic

You may have noticed that I use metaphors and analogies in my practice, where creating meaning from the comparisons helps patients see things from a different yet parallel perspective. It often brings greater clarity to the issue at hand. When I speak about the flexible mindset, I can't help but think of improvisational theater, most often referred to as improv, a form of acting in which most or all of what is performed is unplanned, unscripted, and created spontaneously by the performers.

What actors practice in improv and the skills required to excel at their craft can help establish or rebuild intimacy with your partner. In Katie Goodman's *Improvisation for the Spirit*, she lays out the essential skills required for improvisation or any collaborative and creative process that requires a flexible mindset: stay present, be adaptable, let go of the goal, and gag your inner critic.[9]

From these skills and an adapting attitude, you can let go of the past and move ahead. You can surrender your attachments, such as your notions of sexual perfectionism and how and under what rules and conditions you feel you must perform. You can approach sexual and intimate relationships as improv by letting go of your rules, going with the flow, and trusting that all the ideas and abilities you need are already inside you.

The next stop in our journey for turning down your OC volume level so you can make nice with naughty is the emotion of desire; how our pursuit of the familiar, the stable, the comfortable, and the predictable can choke desire out of our sexual and intimate relationships; and the ways to ignite that flame once again.

---

[9] Goodman, Katie (August 1, 2008). *Improvisation for the Spirit: Live a More Creative, Spontaneous, and Courageous Life Using the Tools of Improv Comedy*, p 115. Sourcebooks. Retrieved from https://www.amazon.com/Improvisation-Spirit-Creative-Spontaneous-Courageous/dp/1402211910/ref=tmm_pap_swatch_0?_encoding=UTF8&qid=1640366625&sr=8-1

EXERCISE: WINNING YOUR TUG-OF-WAR

Let's apply Byron Katie's methodology to observe your thinking and the challenge you may have with your inner critic regarding sexual and intimate relationships. This is the first important step to freeing yourself from the stressful and emotional ways of seeing a situation that your ego has convinced you to believe is true. Begin by isolating one of your specific beliefs about yourself and inspecting that feeling by asking yourself four questions of your inner voice:

My ego's belief:

1. Is it true? (Yes or no. If no, move to question 3.)
2. Can you absolutely know that it's true? (Yes or no)
3. How do you react? What happens when you believe that thought?

4. Whom or what would you be without that thought?

Now, let's deepen your inquiry process by posing "turnarounds," statements that reflect the variations of the opposites of your stressful thought. The goal is to see if one or more turnarounds are just as true or even truer than the stressful thought. Come up with three turnarounds to see which is just as true or truer than what your ego is having you believe:

My ego's belief:

Turnaround 1:

Turnaround 2:

Turnaround 3:

Your mind chatter will be made lighter as you learn how to imaginatively, emotionally, and physically practice thinking and acting differently. You'll develop specific strategies for demystifying the anxieties that are blocking your progress toward what you truly want as a sexual being and how you authentically want to show up in the world.

You'll learn how to change your relationship with anxiety and shift from expending your energy on treating anxiety as an enemy to gathering strength by embracing it as a friend. You could bring anxiety along with you, out of the desert and toward your values, and ultimately have more of what you want—expressing and finding enjoyment in your sexuality.

CHAPTER 4

IGNITING YOUR FIRE OF DESIRE

But warm, eager, living life—to be rooted in life—to learn, to desire, to know to feel, to think, to act.
That is what I want. And nothing less. That is what I must strive for.

— **Katherine Mansfield**

Regaining lost intimacy and desire is the most sought-after request of couples drawn to my practice. A flame that once burnt hot is now barely embers. They want to stoke that fire or know whether it's too late. Being able to let go of the tug-of-war with your ego and its pursuit of safety and security are foundational to reigniting desire.

The bottom line is that if your goal is to experience the spontaneity, passion, eroticism, and mystery that once defined your sexual and intimate relationship, you need to turn down the dial on your overcontrolled pursuit of the familiar, the stable, the comfortable, and the predictable. As I'll share in this chapter, reigniting desire again and keeping it alive begins with you showing up as a sexual being, expressing interest in the sexual needs of your partner, and continuously tending to and fueling the flames of passion and longing.

Fuel + Oxygen = Fire

When couples tell me they experience low sexual desire or have a desire problem altogether, I immediately know something is missing. I'm often drawn to one of my favorite metaphors and ask, *"Fire needs two things to keep it going. What are they?"*

That's right: oxygen and fuel. If a fire has no fuel, it'll burn out, even when oxygen is in ample supply. If a fire has plenty of fuel but no oxygen, the flame will die out as well. Therefore, a healthy *fire of desire* requires both fuel and oxygen. I tell couples who bring their complaint of not being close that the intimacy they're seeking has to be the outcome of something. I tell them that they can't just flip a switch and suddenly become intimate with each other again. You can't just throw big logs onto a dying fire and expect them to catch; you have to begin again with kindling.

From a sexuality standpoint, the fuel that stokes the fire of your longing and yearning for each other are the small, everyday contributions to the relationship, including those unexpected, spontaneous ways of being present and proactively engaged. These small actions communicate that your partner is wanted, valued, and appreciated, especially if that message coincides with the person's preferred way of being loved. *The Five Love Languages* by Gary Chapman frames those five loving ways very well:

- words of affection
- quality time
- receiving gifts
- acts of service
- physical touch[10]

---

[10] Chapman, Gary (January 1, 2015). *The 5 Love Languages: The Secret to Love that Lasts*, pp 37–107. Northfield Publishing Company. Retrieved from https://www.amazon.com/Love-Languages-Secret-that-Lasts/dp/080241270X/ref=sr_1_1?crid=3UIX2WIMM41JJ&keywords=The+Five+Love+Languages&qid=1642625766&sprefix=the+five+love+languages%2Caps%2C108&sr=8-1

It doesn't take a lot of fuel to keep the fire burning; it simply requires that the fuel is steadily applied.

Now, we can have all kinds of fuel, but the fire will still go out without oxygen. In this case, oxygen is the embodied view of yourself as a sexual person—a sexual being deserving of sexual expression and fulfillment that is free of anxiety and fear. The fire of desire in your relationship requires the reclamation of your sexual identity and expression, which may have been extinguished by oppressive and repressive cultural messages about sex and sexuality. Moreover, reclaiming your sexual identity and expression also includes realizing that your sexuality doesn't stop just because you leave the house, nor does it simply cease because you became a mother or father. You're a sexual being 24 hours a day.

However, many things distract us from replenishing our fuel, maximizing our oxygen supply, and stoking the fire for our partners. Life's constant demands combined with our intense drive to excel can drain us OCs of our sexuality. From the children and their routines, to work with its constant demands, to caring for aging parents, to stressing over finances, the fire of desire rarely has a chance to catch a spark. And while it may burn hot for one partner in a relationship who isn't as distracted, it may not burn equally hot for the other who is.

The Desire Discrepancy

Many of my OC patients report that their interest in sex is less than their partner's. This discrepancy can be the source of much consternation in intimate relationships. Usually, the partner who wants sex more often can't understand why their partner doesn't feel the same way. First and foremost, you're not alone.

Low sexual desire and difficulty getting aroused are *the* most common complaints among people looking for help from a sex therapist. Many will initially seek help from a medical provider (e.g., gynecologist, urologist, family doctor) in their quest to relieve their low desire and arousal problem. Rarely are medical issues found, and the good doctors won't pathologize your sexuality and promise a pill for your every ill. Instead, quality medical practitioners will suggest a consultation with a sex therapist who is specifically trained in the relational and psychological factors impacting sexual health.

After her gynecologist completed a full physical exam and found that Linda's tests results were normal, Linda was referred to me. When I met with Linda, she told me that her husband, Todd, has grown increasingly frustrated that they don't have sex much anymore, and that it's now down to only two to three times a year. Linda went on to say she rarely thinks about sex with Todd (or anyone else, for that matter). She said that she doesn't initiate sex and only pacifies her husband from time to time when he comes on to her. Typically, however, Linda either ignores his advances or responds with irritation. When they do have sex, Linda reports struggling with lubrication and feels too embarrassed to use lube; consequently, sex can be uncomfortable. She added that the few times per year when sex happens, it often feels void of physical and emotional pleasure.

Low sexual desire and difficulty getting aroused are common feelings among OC people. Over time, the safety and security they sought in their relationship diminished their feelings of longing and passion for each other. When we start to slow down, we often think that the problem is physical, as Linda did in going to her gynecologist. *"Something must be wrong with my body because it's not performing as it should."*

By focusing on the medical, OCs may inadvertently disregard the contextual factors that negatively impact desire and arousal. In short, they manage their lives quite well and with precision, so it's hard for them to reconcile that their relationships aren't as perfect as everything else in their lives. Thus, some OCs hope for a medical condition that can easily and quickly be fixed, this resolving their low sexual desire. In these cases, the ego deflects OC people's attention away from the often complicated and messy contextual factors that impact desire.

Take John and Jackie's story. They first met during their college years, and although they went to different universities, they managed to get together every weekend and during breaks. They would spend entire weekends in bed enjoying each other's bodies. In the ensuing 12 years, John has become increasingly focused on his career as a middle-school principal. The work demands are overwhelming, and he's notorious for arriving early and staying late. Like a dutiful OC, John pours himself into his work, but in doing so, has neglected Jackie increasingly over the years and allowed the desire he once had for her to burn out.

It came to a head for Jackie recently when John's weekend work retreat was canceled. She saw this as an opportunity to reconnect with him. She simply wanted to know John wanted her and that she was still special to him. When John didn't offer to take advantage of the open weekend, she felt dejected. She told him straight up, *"I'm not sure how much longer I can tolerate the lack of physical and emotional intimacy between us. I wanted you to suggest something special for us to do this weekend since your retreat was canceled. We don't spend much time together. We rarely touch each other. I just don't understand what's going on. I think we should see someone."*

Jackie's plea brought John to attention. He was all too well aware that he lacked desire. He recognized the seriousness of the matter but wasn't willing to be vulnerable enough to share his mutual concern. He never told Jackie he had his testosterone checked, expecting (hoping actually) that low testosterone might play a role in his lack of desire. He was disappointed to learn that his levels were normal.

On top of that, he recognized the contradiction in watching porn and masturbating while disinterested in pursuing sex with Jackie. He, too, wanted answers. Jackie's show of courage by confronting John gave him the courage to confront himself—his inner voice scolding him to protect himself and not expose his vulnerabilities, even to his partner.

Many factors can negatively impact desire within an intimate relationship. However, these three are found to be the most prevalent among most couples: when one of the two partners fails to honor their contract of monogamy; taking your partner's fidelity for granted; and deferring your needs and desires to accommodate those of your partner to the point of sacrificing your own identity. Let's look into each.

The Inherent Risks of Monogamy

For centuries, monogamy has been considered the gold standard for relationshipping. Monogamy provides the predictability, safety, and security that many OCs value. Yet monogamy has inherent risks that couples don't discuss, namely the loss of desire, especially within long-term relationships. However, given the cultural privileging of monogamy, it's hard to reconcile that this dominant institution would have weaknesses. We're told our entire life that monogamy is the best arrangement for couples in love and will help ensure a long, lasting, meaningful, and fulfilling relationship.

As a sex-positive sex therapist, I don't privilege one style of relationshipping over another (e.g., singledom, open relationships, polyamory, monogamish, swinging, and monogamy). I recognize that each has its benefits and costs. The challenge is for each individual and couple to decide which set of plusses and minuses they are willing to live with. However, what is for sure is that many couples report being monogamous but not having sex.

Most OCs choose monogamy because that's the "rule"; it's what's expected as the social norm. Yet monogamy is a contract rarely ever fully discussed and explored between partners. Most of the agreement is assumed. So, when I've determined that a couple has a sexless relationship, I engage in a conversation that tests their understanding of that agreement, as I did with Linda and Todd.

"Are you monogamous?" I asked Linda and Todd. They looked at each other and awkwardly nodded. I continued. "What's the definition of monogamy?"

"Being with one person," answered Linda.

"Being how with one person?" I pressed.

"Sexually," answered Todd.

"That's right," I replied. *"Monogamy is sex with one person. If you're not having sex, and monogamy is 'sex with one person,' then you're not monogamous; you're something else."*

I don't know what that something else is, and it's different for different people, but we have to agree that it's not being monogamous. Sex therapists define a sexless-marriage as one where sex occurs less than once per month, on average. So Linda and Todd's marriage and John and Jackie's where sex occurs two to three times per year is what I would describe as a sexless marriage.

Now, while I don't define what sex means for a couple, I do emphasize that sex isn't limited to penetration alone. There's intercourse and outercourse (e.g., sharing fantasies, mutual masturbation, kissing, massaging, taking showers together). Nevertheless, whatever these couples are doing, it's insufficient to meet their definition of monogamy.

I always tell couples with the complaint that one partner has low sexual desire and difficulty in getting aroused is that it's likely an outcropping of that person's thoughts and emotions and unlikely a medical disorder. If they've chosen monogamy as the governing institution for their relationship, I feel compelled to clarify the rights and responsibilities that go along with the agreement and how one of them may not be living up to their contract with their partner.

The Right and Responsibility of Monogamy

The right of monogamy is primarily this: each of you has a right to enjoy and take pleasure in each other's body in ways that no one else gets to. This right is predicated on the expectation that the person will only get their sexual needs met within the relationship. They've forgone getting needs fulfilled by a coworker, a neighbor, or some anonymous person on an app.

Does this mean that every time your partner wants to have sex, you *have* to have sex? Of course not. Everyone has a right to say no to sex, and each of you must reserve this right. If you could *only* say yes to sex, the yes wouldn't have any meaning. It's precisely your ability to say no that gives the yes its meaning.

However, when the noes outnumber the yeses, it's no wonder that the person on the receiving end of the *"I'm not into it right now"* begins to feel angry, resentful, and bitter. Why? Because there was an agreement that sex would only occur within the relationship, that the option of getting in bed with someone else was taken off the table.

This touches on the responsibility of monogamy, showing interest in the sexual needs of the other. Given that the option of getting sexual needs met elsewhere has been taken off the table for your partner, faithful people will ignore or reject interest from others. Consequently, there's a responsibility to show your partner that you continue to desire them. After all, we all want to feel wanted and special to someone. Nevertheless, relationship problems can remerge when your partner doesn't feel wanted or desired, and they may begin to feel trapped by their contract of monogamy with you.

But let me be clear: we marry or commit to one person for one reason and one reason only. It isn't love; people can love each other without being married. Nor is it about being happy; there are many unhappily committed and married people. The reason we commit and marry is that it makes life easier. Life is easier when you know someone has your back. In other words, commitment is about asking the question, *"What can I do to make your life easier?"* The other side of this coin includes the question, *"What can I do to avoid making your life harder?"* You can see how these two questions relate to conditions that impact desire. A lot of irritation from one's partner restricts fuel for desire, and you fuel desire when you make your partner's life easier. When both couples commit to this mutual practice, the flames can burn hot!

Forced into Celibacy

However, some partners change their mind about monogamy. When one partner defaults to a lack of desire as a reason for their disinterest in sex, they set up a double bind. A double bind occurs when you receive two or more conflicting messages. In the case of a sexless, monogamous relationship, one partner says (1) sex won't happen between us despite the agreement of monogamy, and (2) the other may *not* get their sexual needs met elsewhere. So, for the partner on the receiving end of that double bind to keep their commitment to monogamy, they are forced into celibacy. Here is when the monogamy contract has been broken.

While celibacy is an excellent option for many people, it's a decision one must freely make. It's perfectly acceptable for you to be uninterested in sex; however, it's unacceptable to expect that your partner will also be uninterested in sex. True, many couples live happily together with little or no sex shared between them. They've agreed that their relationship thrives under other forms of non-sexual intimacy. However, these aren't the people who typically come to see me. I only see couples where one or both partners are dissatisfied with the lack of desire and sexual intimacy in their relationship.

Taking Your Partner's Fidelity for Granted

The second factor I find that negatively impacts desire is the concept of "moral hazard." Moral hazard describes how people's behavior changes when they know potential risks are managed by someone or something else. Or said differently, you will make different decisions if you know that you don't have to bear the cost of that decision going badly. For example, homeowners take better care of their property than renters. Renters trust that the landlord will take care of anything that goes wrong. Likewise, people with health insurance use healthcare more than those without health insurance under the expectation that the insurance company will bear the cost.

In their book, *It's Not You, It's the Dishes: How to Minimize Conflict and Maximize Happiness in Your Relationship,* authors Paula Szuchman and Jenny Anderson apply the concept of moral hazard to marriage. They summarize moral hazard as the idea that a lack of future anticipated consequences reduces the urgency to address an issue.[11] Within marriage, it's easy to be distracted by the myriad of life's competing demands and consequently put off investing in the relationship. It's as if the marriage certificate ensures that your partner will be here tomorrow, and so you can put off investing in the relationship today. Unfortunately, there are significant costs to doing so.

By now, you've discovered that I love to use metaphors to convey ideas. So comparable to tending continuously to your fire of desire with fuel (those little things) and oxygen (your sexual being) so the flames of passion don't expire, a healthy garden that produces bountiful fruits and vegetables requires constant care and mindfulness as well. When attended to daily, with enthusiasm and interest, the amount of time and effort needed each day isn't that great. But if the garden is left to its own devices, it will become overgrown with weeds that can suffocate the desired vegetation. Sure, you can go a few days without care and attention, and not much will happen. However, prolonged neglect requires intense work to reverse its downward course, or worse, the garden loses its vitality and interest altogether.

---

[11] Szuchman, Paula & Anderson, Jenny (June 12, 2012). *It's Not You, It's the Dishes: How to Minimize Conflict and Maximize Happiness in Your Relationship*, p. xxii. Random House. Retrieved from https://www.amazon.com/Its-Dishes-originally-published-Spousonomics/dp/0385343957/ref=sr_1_1?crid=1TB6CNIRCUMOZ&keywords=Spousonomics%3A+Using+Economics+to+Master+Love%2C+Marriage%2C+and+Dirty+Dishes&qid=1642695552&sprefix=spousonomics+using+economics+to+master+love%2C+marriage%2C+and+dirty+dishes%2Caps%2C67&sr=8-1&asin=0385343957&revisionId=&format=4&depth=1

You might wonder whether this moral hazard is at play in your relationship. Since you've picked up this book, there's a high probability that it is. Recall Frank and Elizabeth from Chapter 2: the couple who, as athletes, found a strong connection around healthy living. Frank had gained weight, and Elizabeth had struggled to find him attractive. What happened here? Why did Frank stop investing in himself in ways that fueled Elisabeth's desire? The situation of moral hazard helps to provide a possible explanation.

You see, commitment, marriage, and monogamy are like insurance policies designed to protect your relationship by eliminating potential threats such as competition. This insurance leads to the expectation that the partner will be here tomorrow. When you take for granted that your partner will be here tomorrow, you're unlikely to invest today because it can wait—you have more urgent matters needing attention. Unfortunately, this expectation can lead committed couples to invest less into the relationship over time, defaulting to the safety and security of the policy.

In short, there are potential costs to the relationship when one partner isn't behaving in ways intended to maintain the other partner's interest in them. Let me put it this way: are you showing up today in a way that makes it easy for your partner to want to stay? For Frank, the answer is no. He's stopped showing up in the relationship the day he stopped investing in himself in ways that would make it easy for Elizabeth to want to stay. Here's the irony: if their relationship ended, there's a high probability Frank would revert to doing what made Elizabeth attractive to him (e.g., going to the gym, upping his attire, and developing himself in other ways that would increase his attractiveness to others).

Essentially, moral hazard describes the process of taking one's partner's fidelity for granted, which inadvertently communicates that the partner is no longer important or special. Desire begets desire. When you show up as a sexual being in ways that invest in the relationship daily, there's an increased probability that your partner will reciprocate. Sometimes, however, it's less about doing more or giving more of yourself. Many OCs, for example, may have done too much to keep the peace and conform and, in the long run, end up sacrificing essential parts of themselves and negatively affecting their sexuality.

Losing Your Self-Identity

The next factor that may impede desire is selficide. Now, I'm not talking about the act of committing suicide or taking life-threatening selfies and accidentally dying. I'm referring to OCs who compulsively accommodate others, fueled by their desire to be liked and avoid conflict. Remember, OC people have a high sense of social obligation and dutifulness. They're willing to make sacrifices to care for others or do what is regarded as the "right thing to do." In many situations, these are admirable characteristics. However, they might also be carried too far, ultimately costing the OC person their self-identity.

Patrick Thomas Malone, MD and Thomas Patrick Malone, MD, authors of *The Windows of Experience: Moving Beyond Recovery to Wholeness*, introduce readers to the concept of selficide. The Malones write that selficide, the act of dying relationally, psychologically, sexually, and even physically, is far more prevalent than the abrupt ending of life by suicide.[12] Essentially, selficide is a lack of playfulness, an inability to share, a lack of internal integrity, and a fear of choosing a course of action for fear that it might be the wrong one. All of these self-sacrificing manifestations contribute to a person slowly ceasing to be.

---

[12] Malone, Patrick Thomas & Malone, Thomas Patrick (October 1, 1992). *Windows of Experience: Moving Beyond Recovery to Wholeness*, p. 28. Simon & Schuster. Retrieved from https://www.amazon.com/Windows-Experience-Moving-Recovery-Wholeness/dp/0671767070/ref=sr_1_1?crid=2RVKM29I94U4S&keywords=The+Windows+of+Experience%3A+Moving+Beyond+Recovery+to+Wholeness&qid=1642696372&sprefix=the+windows+of+experience+moving+beyond+recovery+to+wholeness%2Caps%2C58&sr=8-1

I simply define selficide as the slow process of cleaving away essential parts of yourself to "go along to get along." Selficide is especially prevalent in contexts where there are pressures to conform (e.g., being the perfect mom, dad, husband, wife, employee, son, or daughter, etc.). As a young man, I found I had cleaved away important parts of myself to go along to get along. I conformed in inauthentic ways out of fear that my authenticity would create conflict. If this concept is applicable, your experience of selficide may differ from my own. Nevertheless, selficide is universally the product of suppressed desire where you have come to believe that your wishes, hopes, needs, and longings don't matter or matter less than those to whom you feel obligated.

In the context of sexuality and intimacy in relationships, you've had to suppress your natural desire to conform to others' expectations. The clear message from your ego was that expressing vulnerability by showing desire wasn't safe—that there could be consequences. For example, those who grew up in the Purity Movement of the 1990s had to quash their desire to comply with church teachings and parental expectations that sex only occurs in marriage; masturbation and fantasizing were also discouraged. Consequently, many felt conflicted about their sexuality or unsure what they wanted sexually. As a result, they suppressed desire out of fear of vulnerability. Desire, though, requires vulnerability, and suppressing your desire out of fear is a slow walk toward selficide and losing your identity as a sexual being.

The Annihilation of Difference

Another side of selficide is deferring to your partner's definition of who you are as a sexual being, and perhaps to their definition of other aspects of your personality as well. It makes me think of the peculiar ways that OC people love. Often unwittingly, OCs love in ways that say, *"I want you to be as I want you to be,"* in essence annihilating any differences between them and their partners.

True love, on the other hand, feels special. It says, *"I want you to be as you want you to be."*

In other words, "acceptance of the other" is how genuine love is expressed. This kind of love acknowledges the other as an autonomous being inherently unpredictable and mysterious. For OCs, however, acceptance of the other can be anxiety-inducing because your partner may have needs, wants, and desires that do not comport to your own.

Conversely, you may find yourself in a relationship where you've felt compelled to meet your partner's definition of who they think you ought to be. While you might keep it together for a while, eventually you begin to cleave away parts of yourself to the point where you wake up one day, if you're lucky, and ask, *"Who the fuck am I?"* If you're here, congratulations! I'm thrilled for you. It's your great awakening.

Here's the irony: if you're asking that question, there's a good chance that your partner is asking the same question of you as well. You see, when you cleave away parts of yourself to "go along to get along," it projects a false self to your partner. They then respond to that false self and unwittingly accept it as your authentic self. They have no reason to believe that it isn't the genuine you. In essence, if they love you, they love only the image that you've unwittingly curated for them.

Over time, however, you may reject this curated image that your partner sees and respond with resentment, anger, and bitterness. Your partner will likely be confused by your behavior since it conflicts with the carefully chosen, overcontrolled image you've crafted and projected for years. Ultimately, this leads to, *"Who's this person I married? They're no longer the person I thought they were."*

Some OCs in a romantic relationship feel pressure to conform to the expectations of their partners. Others demand their partners conform to their expectations to stave off anxiety about the unknown and unpredictable. Recall the story of Julius and Barbara in Chapter 3?

Regardless of when Julius gets aroused, sex between him and Barbara can only happen on Saturdays. Barbara's fixed mindset won't allow distractions during her busy week, so she annihilates any option but Saturday, and Julius conforms to her rules, quashing his impulsive desires. Ironically, it's the unpredictable distractions and acting on impulsive moments that Barbara and Julius need to fuel their desire.

Spontaneous, Responsive, and Contextual Desire

I've talked a lot about desire, and you might still have questions about whether your experience of desire is normal. Let's get some answers for you. First, not everyone experiences desire the same. Second, how you experience desire is perfectly normal. However, this isn't the prevailing message. Culturally speaking, society privileges one kind of desire. It's the *"I can go at the drop of a hat regardless of what's going on around me"* kind of desire. It's the kind of yearning that strikes you by surprise. All of a sudden, you're thinking about sex, and now you want it. It's the desire we see in passionate, explosive love scenes in movies.

Dr. Emily Nagoski, in her book, *Come as You Are: The Surprising New Science that Will Transform Your Sex Life*, terms this type of wanting "spontaneous desire." According to Nagoski, 75 percent of men and 15 percent of women report having spontaneous desire.[13] Unfortunately, the influence of movies, grocery-store magazines, music, and even porn, has done a disservice in convincing everyone that impulse-driven desire is the most prevalent, healthy, normal type of desire. Consequently, you might develop a complex if you don't experience spontaneous desire.

---

[13] Nagoski, Emily (March 2, 2021). *Come As You Are: The Surprising New Science That Will Transform Your Sex Life*, p 11. Simon & Schuster. Retrieved from https://www.amazon.com/Come-You-Are-Surprising-Transform/dp/1982165316/ref=sr_1_1?crid=57WKLTMGA2DD&keywords=come+as+you+are+by+emily+nagoski%2C+ph.d&qid=1642701525&sprefix=come+as+you+are%2Caps%2C84&sr=8-1

Women, in particular, are told that spontaneous desire is the correct and best desire to have. Consequently, women ask themselves, *"Do I want to have sex?"* As a result, they likely find that the "want" isn't there. Spontaneous desire presumes the unmistakable sense of "want." Again, there is no one right desire. Your unique way of experiencing desire is right and perfect for you. You might be wondering, however, *"I don't see myself as having spontaneous desire. What's the alternative?"*

Here, Nagoski defines the second type of desire, which she terms *"responsive desire."* This type of desire is when desire shows up in response to stimulation, meaning something sexy happens, and the body responds. For example, many women and men don't experience a "want" for sex. They don't think about it much and may even have a "take it or leave it" mindset. Responsive-desire folks experience increased desire only *after* sexual intimacy has begun. For these people, the question isn't, *"Do I want to have sex?"* The question is, *"Am I willing to have sex?"*

They recognize that they can't rely on the feeling of "want" because it's likely not present. However, they're responsive to their partner's initiation, and desire builds after sex has started. Responsive desire is just as normal and healthy as spontaneous desire, which is excellent news for the five percent of men and 30 percent of women who experience responsive desire.[14]

I bet your OC trait noticed that the ratios don't add up to 100 percent! You'd be correct, once again. Slightly more than half of the women and about 20 percent of men experience neither spontaneous nor responsive desire. The remaining folks experience "contextual desire," which is dependent on—you guessed it—the context. With this type of desire, environmental factors, including internal psychological states and external circumstances, impact one's felt sense

---

[14] Nagoski (n 13).

of interest and readiness for intimacy.[15] While I'm aware of no empirical evidence to date, I suspect that contextual desire highly correlates with OC temperament. OC people are highly sensitive to contextual factors that can help or hinder desire.

Nagoski uses the metaphor of breaks and accelerators to illustrate how contextual desire works. She explains that breaks are factors that turn off desire while accelerators increase it. Many OCs have strong opinions about what must be present to have sex. For instance, if you have a strong preference that you and your partner should shower before sex, you'll be turned off by an un-showered lover, or you would avoid intimacy if you've not showered. Conversely, you might be turned on by the smell of your partner after they've hit the gym. You might also be particularly turned on by a special cologne or perfume.

If you think that someone (e.g., kids, in-laws, house guests) could hear you or your partner have sex, then you'd be too worried to make noises and have fun. Maybe you can quickly become aroused by fantasizing about your partner or someone else. In a similar vein, you may find it exciting to sense someone wanting you or your partner sexually. Sandra was a client who found that her desire for her wife was piqued only when she had affairs with someone else. When the affairs ended, her desire for her wife declined. In short, contextual desire is a complex interaction of various factors that determine your level of arousal.

For nearly your entire life, you've sought the familiar, the stable, the comfortable, and the predictable. So, you've picked up this book because you want to experience the erotic, the mysterious, the passion, and the thrill of aliveness. You want color back in your life. When the fire of desire has turned into embers, the context (fuel and oxygen) is likely out of balance. Therefore, you (and your partner) must address

---

[15] Ibid, pg. 90.

the contextual factors that inhibit your experience of desire, which includes turning down the volume on your overcontrolledness and claiming your inherent sexual nature and entitlement to experience sexual pleasure.

It also includes acknowledging your partner in loving ways, a topic we will cover in the next chapter. We never grow out of wanting to be seen, heard, and appreciated. You and your partner seek evidence that you and they are wanted and desired. The good news is that you can do things each day to indicate your feelings of love and passion toward your partner—ways of introducing little bits of fuel that feed the fire of desire.

EXERCISE: WHAT IS YOUR DESIRE NARRATIVE?

I incorporate many forms of therapy in my work with couples, and Solution Focused Brief Therapy (SFBT) is one such treatment that works so well in the context of sexual and intimate relationships and fueling desire. SFBT is a solution-oriented, goal-directed approach to therapy that focuses on possibilities and strengths rather than problems, weaknesses, or deficits.

SFBT helps couples focus on those moments, those exceptions when the problem of low sexual desire does not exist, and there is sexual fulfillment and satisfaction. They often find potential solutions embedded within those moments—the very things they desire.

We each have a desire narrative, what we long for in a sexual relationship. For this exercise, ask yourself these questions to unearth what desire means to you. Write them out and interpret them as you would a dream. The more honest you are, the more effective this exercise will be. Ask your partner to do the same and compare notes.

In going through this exercise, you may open that crack in the veneer of your vulnerability a bit more and discover things that are comfortable for you to narrate and experience with your partner. I've found that this exercise itself can fuel a couple's desire for each other.

Describe in detail a time when you experienced intense desire.

What is your greatest sexual fantasy?

What turns you on?

What are you truly seeking in sex?

Which of the Five Love Languages communicate to you most of your partner's affection for you?

CHAPTER 5
DO YOUR EYES LIGHT UP?

When a child walks in the room, your child or anybody else's child, do your eyes light up?
That's what they're looking for.

— Toni Morrison

Every year, those damn holiday party invitations arrive, and every year, Sean is thrown into a mild panic. He's filled with self-criticism that he'll fail to make a great impression and, instead, will make a fool of himself. There's a part of Sean that oscillates between *"I'd rather not go and avoid embarrassing myself,"* and *"My absence will not make a good impression on my boss."*

Moreover, he's all too familiar with this personal ritual when attending these types of events: he'll anxiously walk into the venue, scan the place for possible threats (fearing he doesn't measure up), and look for cues of safety and security. Because he's ultimately compelled to do the "right thing," Sean goes and prays that Tom will be there as well; Tom is a good, safe friend.

Sean wants people to think highly of him, to see him as competent and capable. However, he doesn't realize that his hypervigilance consumes a great deal of his energy and focus, causing him to be less attuned to his body language and what it's communicating to others. His gestures (e.g., flat, unexpressive face; monotone voice; averted gaze) don't demonstrate that he's happy to be with his coworkers, especially José, whom Sean has a crush on. José would never have picked up on Sean's interest given Sean's body language that was signaling, *"I don't want to be here; this isn't a fun time for me."*

In these situations, Sean's OC temperament shows up as being highly cautious to possible threats and preoccupied with finding sources of safety and security. Cognitively though, he's not relaxed, nor is he in a party mood. His intense alertness consumes his thoughts, sucking up considerable energy. Ironically, while his colleagues don't register much enthusiasm for being at the party, they don't exhibit his intense discomfort either.

You see, overcontrolled people are naturally hardwired to see new situations and experiences as possible threats rather than opportunities for something pleasurable to happen. OCs tend to mask their true feelings, especially feelings that they've labeled as weaknesses (e.g., anxiety, depression, insecurity, imposter syndrome) that risk the possibility of rejection from others. Ironically, it's your ability to show up in imperfect ways that add to people's positive perceptions of you. In social psychology, this known as the Pratfall Effect.[16] People considered "superior" by others could become more appealing after committing a small pratfall, because a small mistake would allow others to better humanize them and thus like them more.

A consequence of hiding vulnerability is that you likely feel like you're an outsider in most situations, or that people, in general, don't get you. OCs thus tend to experience higher rates of social isolation and loneliness, which can contribute to psychological distress.

When OCs experience psychological distress, they are prone to wear a neutral face that acts as a thick veil designed to conceal intense

---

[16] Aronson, E., Willerman, B., & Floyd, J. (1966). *The Effect of a Pratfall on Increasing Interpersonal Attractiveness. Psychonomic Science, 4*(6), pp. 227–228. Retrieved from https://psycnet.apa.org/record/1966-05356-001.

feelings, such as anxiety. This is exactly what Sean did. He believed that *"I may be feeling anxious inside, but I have it under control by not showing my anxiety."*

Sound familiar? There are many times in my life when I can recall being very anxious, stressed, or frightened, and my face showed no signs of any of those feelings. In some contexts, this worked to my advantage, though it worked against me in many others.

Here's the deal: the neutral face can be misconstrued as threatening, stand-offish, and aloof. Give it a try. Stand in front of a mirror and form a neutral face where no signs of any expression are present. Relax the muscles in your face. Create some space between your teeth. What do you notice? Not so pleasant and welcoming, is it? The next time you stand in line, pay close attention to those whose faces appear neutral. Does their neutral face elicit feelings of comfort, warmth, or desire? Do the blank faces in the crowd do it for you?

In social situations, a neutral or blank face combined with Low Reward Sensitivity[17] (i.e., low anticipation that something pleasurable is about to occur) can make you appear as if you couldn't care less about being present or being around your partner, family, or friends. This, of course, has an impact on people near you. Others may misperceive your hypervigilance (which is manifested as poor social signaling) as disliking them, which is the opposite of what you want—to be liked.

The neutral face represents one of the primary deficits of an overcontrolled person vis-à-vis social signaling, that is, how you communicate nonverbally to others that they are wanted and accepted. The other is the tendency to be critical as a function of the perceived rules that OCs believe need to be followed, which cause others to feel anxiously aroused from constant scrutiny. So, for the recipient of an OC's body language, it's less about the OC's neutral face and more about their expression that's communicating judgment about what's

---

[17] Lynch (n 1), pp 39-40.

right and what's wrong and needing to follow the rules. Consequently, OC's emotionless expressions often override the intimacy of their relationships by never allowing what they may feel in their hearts to show in their eyes.

I remember when I first learned about the effects of a person's neutral face and hypervigilance on another through my favorite TV program growing up: *The Oprah Winfrey Show*. I loved Oprah's show. I watched it every day after school. I loved peering into the private lives of others and seeing how other families were also as complex as my own family, and often more so. One particular episode in Oprah's *Life Class Series* that stands out for me is when she interviewed Toni Morrison, who had just released *The Bluest Eye*, her first novel. In the interview, Ms. Morrison said, *"When a kid walks in the room—your child or anybody else's child—does your face light up? That's what they're looking for."*

The author went on to describe how when her young children walked into the room, she approached them, not with an eye of enthusiasm but with an eye of criticism: *"Were their pants buckled? Were their hair combed? Were their socks pulled up?"* She then described how she rationalized her approach. She sincerely thought that her love and affection were on display as a caring and concerned mom, but now recognizes that all her children saw was that *"my critical face looked for problems."*

Morrison then shared her epiphany, saying that from then on, she learned to let her face speak what was in her heart because, when her children walked into the room, she sincerely was happy to see them. That genuine feeling was directly from her heart, and she wanted that message to shine through for them.[18]

---

[18] Oprah's Lifeclass (May 26, 2000). *"Does Your Face Light Up?"* Oprah Winfrey Network. Retrieved from https://www.youtube.com/watch?v=9Jw0Fu8nhOc.

Oprah considers this one of the biggest lessons of her show in the 1990s. As she describes it, *"The common denominator in the human experience is that everybody first wants to be appreciated and validated and that children value themselves based on others' reactions."*[19] Our face helps to communicate this love.

Here's your takeaway: we never grow out of wanting to be seen, heard, and appreciated. In the context of sexuality or intimacy, you and your partner want evidence that you and they belong together and are desired. Let me ask you then: when your partner walks into the room, do your eyes light up? Sure, you may have opinions about how they appear, but do you look past that to find the good in them? *"It's so good to see you. I'm glad you're home. How was your day?"* When your partner enters the room, do you turn off the TV or turn the sound down completely to honor their presence, or do you barely acknowledge them? Does your smartphone or tablet get more face time than they do?

A Blank Face Misspeaks Volumes

There's an old saying in my profession: "One cannot *not* communicate." Even when we're uninvolved relationally, our partners are still unconsciously picking up messages from us. So, although we may think we aren't communicating, we still are. Sadly, though, we often communicate unintended messages. How often have you said to someone, *"Well, that wasn't my intention,"* as you then try to explain your intention?

One evening, my partner and I made dinner and decided to watch a movie. We have an earlier model smart TV, which means I need to use the Bluetooth technology on my laptop to stream HBO Max onto the television screen. So here I am intensely concentrating on how to

---

[19] ibid.

connect my computer to the TV while my partner, having partially undressed, begins playfully dancing to show off her new panties.

Where's my attention? Sure, I noticed what she was doing, but my attention was dedicated to the task at hand: to get the TV to sync up with the computer. Unfortunately, my expressionless, neutral face communicated to her that I was annoyed by her, which wasn't how I felt at all. As a result, she became upset with me. When my partner started dancing, she wanted to be seen, and my eyes didn't light up. I allowed my rule of *"I have to get this technology synced for me to proceed to the next thing on the agenda"* to override what was more important, which was to take advantage of a fun, spontaneous moment together.

Your Behavior Is Where You Begin

In Chapter 1, I shared how my college professor's review of my training tapes prompted his feedback that I had perfected the psychoanalytic poker face. I struggled with how to listen intensely while nonverbally communicating warmth and caring. Yet despite my desire to communicate kindness and empathy, my intense focus on understanding my clients' experiences overrode that desire. Consequently, my patients were left feeling insecure and wondering what I was doing with the personal information they were sharing with me.

Research shows that neutral, expressionless faces, much like my poker face, are frequently interpreted as hostile or disapproving and can trigger an automatic defensiveness in people.[20] Now, of course, a flat facial expression emotionally affecting another person also depends on context. A neutral face is less likely to be seen out of context in

---

[20] Butler EA, Egloff B, Wilhelm FH, Smith NC, Erickson EA, Gross JJ. (March 3, 2003), *The Social Consequences of Expressive Suppression*. Emotion Journal.10.1037/1528–3542.3.1.48. PMID: 12899316. Retrieved from https://pubmed.ncbi.nlm.nih.gov/12899316/.

situations where subdued expressions of emotion are expected, for instance, at a funeral or when negotiating a business deal.

Conversely, a poker face can be very disconcerting and easily misinterpreted by others in situations where you would normally expect expressions of emotions, such as when you're on a date or when arguing with your partner. In the case of Sean, his expressionless *"I don't want to be here"* body language at the party completely confounded someone he genuinely desired to be with, José.

This book is all about reclaiming yourself as a sexual being, and the information I'm sharing in this chapter is intended to help you notice how you show up when you're with your partner. Observing yourself in context and, most importantly, owning what you're communicating regardless of your intentions puts you in the center lane on the road to making nice with naughty.

Putting the Flames Behind the Eyes

Let's begin with the title of this chapter. Our eyes lighting up communicates warmth and enjoyment in having the other person in our presence. You might ask, *"Yeah, but what does it mean to have your eyes light up?"* Simply put, it means slightly raising your eyebrows, smiling gently, and softening the eyes.

Raised eyebrows, also known as the "eyebrow wag," communicate interest, empathy, and affection. Thomas R. Lynch, the founder of Radically Open Dialectical Behavior Therapy, whom I introduced in Chapter 1, defines "eyebrow wag" as a universal social acceptance signal involving a concurrent upward movement of both eyebrows, most often accompanied by an authentic smile, happy eyes, and an agreeable tone of voice. He goes on to say that eyebrow wags are a natural way of saying, *"I like you"* or *"you are in my tribe."*[21]

---

[21] Lynch (n 1), p 162.

Eyebrow wags signal interest to the other person, as well as willing intentions and openness, and receptivity to new information or critical feedback. Lynch says that raised eyebrows are noticeably absent when we're greeted by someone who dislikes us. However, in terms of an OC's temperament, a blank face with no raising of eyebrows isn't always associated with dislike. OCs rarely exhibit eyebrow wags. Their intention isn't to communicate that they dislike everyone; it's more likely that they're creating a psychological distance in response to their hypervigilance.

Now that I've shared this with you, during the coming days, pay attention to the position of your eyebrows when you greet or talk with your partner. Are they high to communicate pleasure, or are they low or furrowed (assuming no Botox® injections) to express criticism or worry? You might now be saying to yourself, *"Yeah, but if I'm thinking or worried about something, why would I want to fake it with a happy face?"*

Great question. Let's examine if it's "faking it." You can still be concerned about something—like being super-focused on getting a movie to play—while still being open to novel, unexpected experiences, such as one's partner playfully dancing in front of you. A simple eye wag that says, *"I see you. I like you. You're more important than what I'm doing right now"* can go a long way.

However, notice my mind chatter at the time: *"Yeah, but we had an agreement that we would finish up dinner and watch a movie together. It's my job to get the TV synced to the computer. Without this pivotal step, the plans are ruined."* Can you see the embedded rules and the fixed-mindset?

Recall the sky and clouds metaphor from Chapter 3. You are the sky, the sentinel of your entire being, and your thoughts and feelings are the clouds that form your mind chatter. Even though these thoughts and feelings that you're observing may appear convincing, they don't define your experience and govern your behavior. It's the same as Toni Morrison learning to let her *"love and affection face"* communicate her feelings toward her children, overriding her intense focus on social rules about appearance.

In the same vein, I suspect you want your partner to be seen, validated, and felt desired by you, right? Here's where you can acknowledge the clouds and redirect your attention toward behaviors that reflect your values, such as having your eyes light up when they enter the room. Ultimately, you're not being fake when you're living by your values.

Secondly, your intentional eye-raises, even if "simulated," activate neuroregulatory systems that are bi-directional, meaning that these behaviors can trigger positive feelings within you, as well as positive emotions within your partner. Once you have the "eyebrow raise" comfortably added to your repertoire of communicating, you're now ready to incorporate some other forms of body language that can stoke the flames of desire between you and your partner.

To that end, there are three ways of being present and active in your sexual and intimate relationships:

- cognitively, by getting your mental groove back;
- being an emotionally available lover; and
- by getting physical.

Although there is overlap, let's explore each separately and discover the tools you can use to be more adaptive and in the moment with your partner.

Getting Your Mental Groove Back

Everything we're talking about in this chapter came naturally to you as a baby, such as raising your eyebrows when a family member walked into the room, or what we'll cover shortly, deep and relaxed stomach breathing and having fun pretending without feelings of faking it.

Babies are exclusively belly breathers. Unfortunately, they become chest breathers over the course of their lives. Children are also naturally un-self-conscious until they develop an ego and a sense of "Me, My, Mine," and all hell breaks loose. In sexuality and intimacy, OC people have a love/hate relationship with pretending. They want sex to feel "natural," and if it doesn't, then something's wrong. OCs are very sensitive and actively on guard for anything they deem as wrong. If they're feeling anxious, then something's wrong, or if their partner wears a strap-on dildo or uses a lube, that's not natural and therefore wrong.

You have to get back into the groove of understanding that "pretending" is not wrong. At the very least, it can be your communication to your partner that you are present. At the very most, it can send them a message that you're in the playground and ready to make nice with naughty, as my partner tried to do earlier in the chapter and I missed her communiqué completely.

Being present as a sexual being begins with you declaring that you are, in fact, a sexual being. You've always been one and will always be; it's your nature. Sure, there's a lot that has contributed to you dampening your sexual expression, but it's still there, hidden within you. No doubt you've beaten yourself up for your lack of desire, especially given your rate of success in all other aspects of your life. You now want to attain the holy grail of a satisfying intimate and sexual relationship. I'm with you! Many OCs, as mentioned before, have been conditioned out of their sexuality, and it's time you get your groove back.

Cheryl Fraser's *Buddha's Bedroom: The Mindful Loving Path to Sexual Passion and Lifelong Intimacy* is a sexually playful guide containing mindfulness exercises, sex therapy techniques, and Buddhist teachings to help couples spark passion in their relationships.[22] What's required

---

[22] Fraser, Cheryl Ph.D. (January 2, 2019). *Buddha's Bedroom: The Mindful Loving Path to Sexual Passion and Lifelong Intimacy*, p 20. Reveal Press. Retrieved from

in Fraser's approach is that true passion is sustainable if you're willing to shift your perspective from *"my partner is the problem"* to your own mind being the problem. She adds that you must take responsibility for your passion and get active about it (that's job #1) because *you* are the critical driver to passion in your relationship, not someone else.

Triangular Theory of Love

Passion is an essential ingredient to a meaningful and fulfilling relationship. When I talk with couples about each wanting to be loved and desired by the other, I often find it helpful to break down the elements that comprise an intimate and loving relationship using Dr. Robert J. Sternberg's *Triangular Theory of Love*. His theory proposes that love can be understood in terms of three components, each of which represents different aspects of love: commitment, intimacy, and passion.[23] For the purposes of this book, I arranged the three elements from the easiest for OCs to manage, "commitment," to the hardest, "passion."

The Triangle of Love

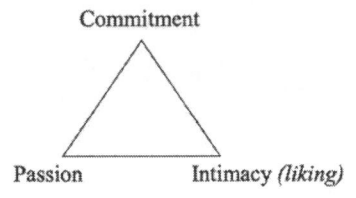

Commitment

Passion　　　　Intimacy *(liking)*

Commitment refers to the decision to love a certain other and stay connected to that other person to fulfill the "until death do us part"

---

https://www.amazon.com/Buddhas-Bedroom-Mindful-Lifelong-Intimacy/dp/1684031184.

[23] Sternberg, R. J. (1986). *A Triangular Theory of Love. Psychological Review, 93*(2), pp 119–135. Retrieved from https://doi.org/10.1037/0033-295X.93.2.119.

vow in a marriage. As I shared in Chapter Four, we often marry or commit to one person for one reason only, and it isn't love or happiness. People can love each other without being married, and there are many unhappily committed and married people. The primary benefit of commitment and marriage is that it makes life easier by providing safety and security. As you might imagine, OCs tend to emphasize commitment and find it relatively easy to do. However, commitment without intimacy and passion can make for an empty form of love.

I should note here that some OCs, especially OC men, find that they can have affairs independent of how they may feel about their spouse and still feel committed to their spouse and have no desire to leave them. They want the safety and security of their partner, so they stay committed.

Intimacy, according to Sternberg, refers to feelings of closeness, connectedness, and bondedness in loving relationships, of which many couples enjoy an over-abundance. They'll often say to me, *"We make for great friends."* Now, keep in mind that Sternberg uses the term *intimacy* differently than I have in previous chapters. Here, Sternberg refers to intimacy as "liking" each other. In this framework, liking and commitment form what can be termed "Companionate Love."

Many couples who come to see me say that they're friends with each other. They see themselves as companions, roommates essentially. Their intimacy element is solely found in the friendship quality of their relationship. They've accepted living together in a passionless relationship primarily for safety and security's sake. Many OCs find they're committed to each other and may even like each other, but something vital remains adrift and increasingly floating out of reach. They lack passion.

Passion refers to the physical attraction and sexuality in loving relationships. Passionate love and intense sexual attraction and desire are what we often feel for one another at the beginning of a relationship; it's what many describe as infatuation. Passion burns hot, and it can disappear just as suddenly. To sustain a relationship, commitment and intimacy (or liking) need passion. Unfortunately, it's the most common element in short supply among OC couples.

Passion necessitates a willingness to have playful moments unencumbered by mind chatter. These moments may also include playful pretending. To express passion, one must act courageously in ways that might garner rejection from your partner. In the context of sexuality or intimacy, it may help to look upon your courage and mindfulness as a lighthouse guiding your thoughts and actions.

Even when you have a tempest of clouds and storms around you, you're still able to move continuously toward your guiding light. All of your efforts are aligned in that direction and convey your desire for intimacy for your partner and yourself.

Your beliefs and desires need to be communicated to your partner to override your acceptance of "moral hazard" that we discussed in Chapter 3: the notion that you don't have to worry about communicating your desire because your partner is going to understand your blank face or peer behind your furrowed brows and assume the love is there. That's not the solution; the only solution is you showing up as a sexual being and taking care of it yourself.

Communicate from your heart and not your head. For the triangle of love to be in balance—what Sternberg refers to as "Consummate Love"—you need a balance of all three components: commitment, intimacy, and passion working together toward an ideal relationship. You constantly have to stoke the fire of desire with new fuel, and with your presence to provide the much-needed oxygen.

Being an Emotionally Available Lover

The second way of showing up as a sexual being is by being emotionally available, open, and receptive to your partner, and communicating that you are present and desire them. OCs have been working that hypervigilance muscle for a long time and are often unaware of its command over their true selves. In the story above, Sean arrived at the party as not relaxed or in a party mood because of his intense alertness. It drained him emotionally and prevented his true self from showing up.

According to Thomas Lynch, there are five broad classes of emotion identified as "cues," each reflecting the result of a natural selection process that equips us to attend to and respond to certain types of situations. In the context of sexual and intimate relationships, each situation describes a visceral emotion in us, and each communicates a different message to others.[24]

Social Safety Cues are associated with being included and part of a group. When our safety cues are activated, we experience a sense of calm and contentment and a desire to associate with others. We're more open and playful and more curious about the world. Our bodies are relaxed, our breathing is calm and deep, and our hearing is enhanced. A little later in the chapter, you'll discover how to create contentment and desire, so safety cues can allow you and your partner's fire of desire to burn.

Novelty Cues are unexpected experiences or events that trigger an immediate evaluation process to determine if the cue is essential for our well-being. When these cues are activated, our bodies are frozen in place, and breathing is suspended or up in our chest. We're alert, but we're not aroused as we evaluate the new experience. If we consider the novel experience safe, we return to our sense of contentment and communicate our calmness and readiness through our eyes, body language, and tone of voice.

Tomeka and Niko recently came in to see me about the loss of passion in their relationship. Tomeka described how she would start being sexual with Niko by undressing him in front of the living room

---

[24] Lynch (n 1), pp 37–41.

window. It's erotic for her. However, Niko immediately began to worry that neighbors might see them, which would be mortifying. Apparently, the odds of the neighbors seeing Tomeka and Niko were rather slim. It was light outside and dark inside. Nevertheless, Niko experienced the situation as a threat because he didn't feel safe in the novelty of the moment. Of course, Tomeka felt rejected, too, which caused a chill in the room for some time.

Rewarding Cues are experiences that we evaluate as potentially gratifying. We expect that something pleasing is about to happen. Our bodies are energized and awash with feelings of well-being. Our breathing and heart rate are faster as we anticipate something enjoyable will happen to us. We become excited, even passionate about receiving the experience.

Rewarding cues can also elicit hyper-goal-focused behavior that can negatively impact those around us and cause us to neglect how they may be reacting to us through their vocal cues and facial expressions. Examples of this are diving into your dinner before everyone else is served or dominating a conversation because you're so excited about what you have to share.

Threatening Cues are stimuli that we've determined to be potentially dangerous or harmful to us. When we feel threatened, we anticipate that something terrible will occur or our goals may be blocked. Our sympathetic nervous system is activated, triggering feelings of anxiety and an urge to flee or detach ourselves from the experience or stay present and challenge or attack it. It's the old flight or fight response being activated. Our bodies feel tense, sweaty, and agitated. We get goosebumps, our breathing becomes shallow, and our hearts pump faster.

Overwhelming Cues are the extreme of threatening cues, which can trigger an evolutionary, older emergency shutdown system needed for survival. Rewarding cues can have the same shutdown effect if they continue unabated or increase in intensity. Our heart rate, breathing, and body movements slow down considerably because our safety system and our threatening system are disabled. We lose all facial expressions and appear numb, unresponsive, and insensitive to pain.

While safety, novelty, and rewarding cues are most associated with positive sexuality and intimacy in relationships, it sometimes makes perfect sense to be sensitive to threatening and overwhelming cues. There's a degree of protection from that focus, and the results can be gratifying. In other words, if you prevent a catastrophe, the payoff is enormous. It's equivalent to being diligent about preventative maintenance on your car. It's so rewarding hearing your mechanic say, *"I noticed a tiny crack in your engine block. It's a good thing you brought it in when you did because that could have been a disaster on the highway."*

Being highly sensitive to threatening and overwhelming cues has been worthwhile for us OCs across many areas of our lives. They're so rewarding that they've become our primary focus, driving and commanding our emotions, unfortunately to extremes that cloud our vision and hurt our relationships. As in Sean's story earlier, his feeling threatened and ultimately overwhelmed by his environment caused him to avoid engaging with others or even being in tune with the feelings of others.

Getting Physical

The third way of showing up as a sexual being is physical. Although defining it as *behavioral* may be more accurate, *physical* is more appropriate in this context. The body often follows the mind in terms of the neuropathways activated. For instance, when we light up our eyes, smile, or breathe deeply from our stomachs, those physical actions release feel-good hormones. Even if you're not in a particularly jovial mood, you're tapping into pleasant hormones by showing up just a little more physically. This is akin to the improv techniques I described earlier, where you're showing up as an actor, wanting your acting partner to have a natural and spontaneous response to your response by saying *"yes, and"* instead of *"yes, but."*

The OC person tends to be someone others would describe as tightly wound. Because they are so high functioning, they're inclined to take on a tremendous amount of responsibility and tend to be quite tense and anxious, as a rule.

This understanding of the five emotions can be helpful in folding down the porcupine quills of an OC's intense alertness to threatening and overwhelming cues so that they can start cooling their nervous system and create a context to enjoy the novelty and reward cues more conducive to sexual and intimate relationships.

Take a Breath

A common complaint among many OCs is that they often feel tense, which is partly due to their tendency to take on a lot of responsibility (out of fear that others won't do a good enough job). Yes, I'm talking to you here! Consequently, you're stressed, and stress is a real desire killer for many. One way to help alleviate the stress and cool down your nervous system is through breathing exercises. Breathing exercises take little effort but have huge payoffs.

Let's take a moment to engage in an exercise that I use in my practice. Sit, resting comfortably against the back of the chair. Put one hand on your belly and the other on your chest and breath regularly. Observe your hand and shoulder movements. Which hand moves the most: the lower hand or the upper hand? Do your shoulders seem to rise and fall with each breath? If your upper hand moves and shoulders rise and fall, you're likely a chest breather.

If you've also subconsciously got into the habit of keeping your stomach tight, you've probably acquired chest breathing as well. If anything, chest-breathing stokes anxiety, not desire. OC people are notoriously chest breathers. They can hold a lot of anxiety in their chest. (If you want to give yourself a panic attack, try rapid, shallow chest breathing for 60 seconds…on second thought, don't do that!)

Instead, let's try belly breathing. Once again, place one hand on your belly and one on your chest. Try to pull the breath down to your navel this time, slowly counting to five, pushing the lower hand out while the upper hand and chest remain still. Do this for 60 seconds. What did you notice? Many people find deep cleansing breaths feel calming and can dampen anxiety. Those clouds begin to float out of sight.

Now, some OCs find that this style of deep breathing itself triggers anxiety. They find their minds filled with thoughts such as, *"This is a waste of time."* or *"Am I even doing it right?"* and *"Jeez! Sixty seconds seem like FOREVER. I got shit to do!"* Each one of these thoughts is just another cloud. Notice them without judgment. You'll likely find your feelings shifting toward a calmer state. Moreover, just as eyebrow raises release positive hormones, deep breathing can calm your nerves and reduce your stress. From this improved state, imagine being more flexibly open to desire.

In the coming days and weeks, practice maximizing the positive effects of deep breathing. Begin to notice if you're holding tension in your belly or shoulders. Allow the tension to be the signal for you to relax your stomach and lower your shoulders. You might find that you'll do this multiple times a day. However, as the days progress, you'll find that it becomes more automatic.

You'll find yourself interacting with people with greater energy and openness from this more relaxed state. The breathing exercise essentially allows your parasympathetic nervous system, your body's rest and digestion response, to take charge, calming you down, reducing your stress, and enabling you to approach your partner differently.

Even if it feels awkward and unnatural in the beginning —and it probably will be because you're not used to it— wanting your partner to feel desired and your own need to feel desired will override your sense of unnaturalness. Those thoughts are ginned up by your ego defending itself from the uncertainty and risk inherent in feelings of desire and passion. Stick with this exercise. You'll find yourself unconsciously breathing more and more from your stomach, for you'll be in alignment with your true values and desire for your partner.

Build a Campfire Together

Here's another metaphor I often use, inspired by the practice of BDSM (Bondage/Discipline, Dominance/Submission, Sadism/Masochism). Some BDSM scenes might involve physical restraints, the granting and relinquishing of control, and the infliction of pain. These activities are performed among mutually consenting relationships that emphasize informed consent. BDSM participants have a concept called "safe, sane, and consensual" that provides the minimum sense of safety and security that allows participants to feel close and intimate.

Now, many people, upon reading my material or hearing me speak, might assume that I'm suggesting closeness is deleterious to relationships because of its components of low risk, low anxiety, and high predictability. That isn't the case at all. What I'm saying is that closeness—in the absence of intimacy or as a substitute for intimacy—is an unspoken contract with your partner to be passionless roommates. I also believe that, in the context of safe, sane, and consensual, the "closeness" element achievable through that consent creates balance and allows passion and expressions of desire to flame up within the structure of those agreements.

It's similar to building a campfire (what I term a "love fire" in the exercise that follows). Fire is inherently unpredictable, so the rocks you place around the fire pit represent the safe, sane, and consensual agreements that allow the fire to burn with minimal hypervigilance. They allow you to be spontaneous and unpredictable within the safety of the circle of rocks and enable you and your partner to make nice with naughty in a sort of mutually agreeable and controlled environment.

Passion begins with you. Presumably, in picking up my book, you felt a sense of something missing. You felt inhibited in your ability to have fulfilling and satisfying sexual and intimate relations with your partner. Your temptation as an OC has been to attribute your dissatisfaction to the context of the moment: *"I can't get hard,"* or *"he hasn't showered,"* or *"we're not supposed to have sex during the week,"* and on and on. But you're not going to accept that fate any longer. Are you?

It begins with you treating your partner with the assumption that passion is already there and that you can undoubtedly stoke those embers. It's you living out the Solution Focused Brief Therapy exercise that you and your partner completed in the previous chapter. That practice was designed to open that crack in the veneer of your vulnerability a bit more and discover things that are comfortable for you to narrate and experience with your partner. It's very similar to the exercise that you and your partner will engage in at the end of this chapter by building a campfire—what we'll call a "love fire"—together.

Remember, my intent is not to turn overcontrolled people into under-controlled people. UCs don't need to have rocks around their campfire. They don't care if the fire burns out of control and spreads outside its circle. Instead, I intend to help you turn down the dial on your overcontrolledness and let the fire of desire do what it naturally does within a context that allows you to enjoy it. Without the rocks, the fire would feel too intense and uncontrollable. However, by building a campfire with your partner and choosing and placing rocks together, you both can create a safe, sane, and consensual experience where passion can burn.

EXERCISE: BUILDING A LOVE FIRE TOGETHER

In this exercise, I would like you and your partner to build a love fire together on your bedroom dresser or nightstand. Don't worry, you're not going to light it literally, but you will figuratively.

As with a campfire, you'll need to create a fire pit for your love fire. The first step I want you and your partner to take is to collect six or eight (or more) rocks, each roughly the size of an avocado. Yes, I want you to physically gather and build stuff for this exercise. Remember, you're both cultivating passion between you, so consider making a meaningful adventure of it by driving together to a local brook or stream or an open field to find some rocks and experience doing this exercise together.

I often ask my patients to go even further and collect small twigs and cut slivers of yellow and red construction paper to place inside the rock circle to resemble a real fire.

The next step is for you and your partner to write a word or phrase on each rock describing the safe, sane, and consensual agreements that will allow you to express your passion for each other. Safety cues could be words such as:

Kindness	Trust	Communication
Quiet	Boundaries	Sharing
Fun	Support	Selflessness
Respect	Commitment	Empathy

What you write down on each stone in a visible color are those things that reflect your values and are important to you. The words or phrases you choose will allow you to be spontaneous and unpredictable within the safety of the circle of rocks and enable you to make nice with naughty in your mutually agreeable and controlled environment.

The most important step throughout this exercise is showing up as a sexual being to provide the oxygen—the embodied view of yourself as a person deserving of sexual expression and fulfillment—free of anxiety and fear, and open and accepting of the reward of intimacy you and your partner both desire and deserve.

CHAPTER 6
LETTING YOUR VALUES GUIDE YOU

"Remember that wherever your heart is, there you will find your treasure. You've got to find the treasure so that everything you have learned along the way can make sense."

— Paulo Coelho

Steve, a 47-year-old corporate executive, loved Terry very much. They lived together for more than 15 years. They had a lot going for them. Both were very satisfied with their careers and enjoyed their leisure time, including being exceptional travel partners. Yet something was missing. The vitality of their sexual desire for each had withered away over the years and simply died.

They were merely glorified roommates for more than a third of their relationship. Before entering their sexual desert, sex between them had occurred intermittently. But for the past five years, there was nothing. For a while, Terry tried to get Steve excited and occasionally pursued him sexually at night while they lay in bed together.

Steve, however, would respond by tightening up his entire body and becoming rigid. He'd feel anxious inside as well, which led him to become angry and agitated, both at himself and the situation Terry put him in. It caused Steve to emotionally and physically push Terry away.

By all accounts, Steve and Terry loved each other. They enjoyed their time together and were great friends. They knew and accommodated each other so well, which is what made their travel adventures so enjoyable. Steve judged himself harshly for not having the kind of sexual desire that mirrored Terry's interest. (Terry, in the meantime, had stopped initiating sex after his many failed attempts.) Steve intuited that the passion wasn't there anymore and was becoming increasingly pessimistic that there would be an oasis in their sexual desert where a satisfying and meaningful sexual relationship could be found.

Steve had tried psychotherapy before. He was confident that this was about him and not about Terry. He needed to figure this out because he didn't want to lose his life partner. However, Steve felt too embarrassed to discuss his sex life with his prior therapists. To do so seemed too private and would leave him feeling vulnerable.

This time felt different, however. Steve found himself to be more eager and willing. It was as if something was guiding him out of his desert. Something more meaningful. Moreover, the prospect of losing Terry meant too much to him.

When Steve came to see me, we reviewed his sexual history up until the current moment. I immediately hooked onto the spark of enthusiasm that was pulling him toward entering therapy once again. We began to process the parts of him that reflected his ideal self—the person he wanted to be in the world and how he wanted to be with Terry again. We began talking about Steve's values, those qualities at the core of his being, now guiding him through his desert to a more sexually satisfying and intimate relationship with Terry.

Our North Star

Our values provide us with clues as to what actions to take in our lives when things become uncertain and stressful. Values aren't destinations; that would be viewing values the wrong way. Instead, they support our movement toward what's important to us and guide us in our attempts to live authentic lives. In other words, values are our North Star. Even with the desert terrain being flat, featureless, unpredictable, and poorly lit, you have your North Star to guide you, to help you determine what actions to take, in what direction to place your foot—in this moment—and move on that bearing toward your special destination.

Moreover, just as with the North Star, no matter how far you travel, how much time you invest in getting there, or the amount of effort you exert, you'll never arrive at the North Star. Similarly, values guide you toward your aspirational—the person you want to be—by helping you identify the actions that support your progress toward what you truly want and how you authentically want to show up in the world. Yet you have to accept that you will never arrive at being your ideal self; you will never be "finished" as a perfect human being.

Let's say one of your values is kindness; after all, OCs tend to be very conscientious people. Consequently, you want your behaviors to reflect that of a kind person. While you're driving to the grocery store, you see a panhandler at the intersection. You decide to roll down your window and hand them a five-dollar bill. Have you now concluded your pursuit of kindness? Does this mean that you can check this off of your "to-do" list and never have to be kind again? No, of course not. You continue to do things that are kind because doing kind things reminds you of what's important to you—kindness—and that you're living out a value that's of importance to you and how you engage with the world.

In this chapter, I apply the concept of values to the context of making nice with naughty, to help you gain clarity on what's important to you vis-à-vis your sexual behavior. Many people talk about values but seldom define them; I do and offer them as guideposts to living that authentic life. Every step of the way, I'll invite you to take a look at whether your sexual and intimate behaviors reflect your values.

For example, the words you wrote on your rocks in the last exercise are your and your partner's values. They're shared values because you both chose and encircled those rocks to create a desire-fire pit where passion for each other can burn freely. Values reflect your deepest desires for how you want to behave and interact with others, for what matters most to you, and for what you want to represent. They guide and motivate your actions in your relationships and represent the kind of partner you continuously aspire to be.

Given how important values can be in your ability to experience and express your sexuality, it's helpful to distinguish values from your achievements, your beliefs, and your feelings. Knowing the difference can make all the difference in your ability to show up as the sexual being you're meant and truly desire to be.

What Values Are and Are Not

To explore values personally, let's begin by defining what they are in the general sense. In their book, *Acceptance and Commitment Therapy for Couples*, Avigail Lev and Matthew McKay give guidance about what values are and are not—to encourage values-guided, mindful action between couples.[25]

In my practice, I like to use their seven delineations of the concept of values to distinguish what values are and are not in the context of making nice with naughty. I apply that structure to help couples think through how they want to be with each other and what specific changes they're willing to make. Use these seven distinguishing characteristics to take action based on your values and open yourself to greater intimacy and enrichment in your sexual and intimate relationships.

---

[25] Lev, Avibail, PsyD & McKay, Matthew, PhD. (March 1, 2017). Acceptance and Commitment Therapy for Couples: A Clinician's Guide to Using Mindfulness, Values, and Schema Awareness to Rebuild Relationships, pp 51–3. Context Press. Retrieved from https://www.amazon.com/Acceptance-Commitment-Therapy-Couples-Relationships/dp/162625480X/ref=sr_1_3?crid=1PQEZAQ4YVYRO&keywords=acceptance+and+commitment+therapy+for+couples&qid=1645454865&sprefix=acceptance+and+commitment+therapy+for+couples%2Caps%2C69&sr=8-3.

1. Values Are Not Goals

Overcontrolled people are highly conscientious people. We strive to do the right thing, be honest, live with integrity, and be fair to others. However, OCs can have difficulty distinguishing goals from values and often live out their values as if they were goals.

OC people tend toward perfectionism and emphasize goals and outcomes as evidence of their competency. Having the objective clear in their minds makes them feel successful only if they achieve those objectives. *"Am I sexy/attractive enough?" "Will I satisfy my partner?" "Will I get an erection?" "Will I even want to have sex?"* However, goals can also trigger psychological obstacles, especially when OCs lack confidence in achieving their goals *and* believe that their worth is tied to achieving them as well.

For example, Will worries about ejaculating too soon. He thinks to himself, *"I'm so afraid that I won't be able to satisfy my partner because I'll come before her."* As with so many OCs, Will's mind has a picture of what "sex should look like," and he's conscientious, too, of his partner's needs and wants. Consequently, he worries that he'll fail to meet his objective of pleasuring his partner, which triggers his feelings of inadequacy and emasculation. You can already imagine how the confusion between values and goals can trigger his avoidance of sex, which his partner can misperceive as a lack of interest in sex. It isn't that Will lacks interest in sex; he lacks interest in experiencing a reoccurrence of shame, embarrassment, and humiliation that's become associated with sex.

Goals reflect the outcomes or the destination based on a series of actions. But how do you decide what steps to take? As the saying goes, "All roads lead to Rome." Which road(s) do you take? Your answer sources from your particular preferences. The goal is getting to Rome, but the path you choose is based on what's important to you—your values.

Values are essentially your ideal view; they inspire you. They're always something that you strive for and constantly work toward, even if you never achieve them. The pursuit keeps the value alive in you and keeps you on the right path with the right mindset. As example, pleasure-based sex is a value, not a goal. Even when sex doesn't happen the way you want it to (you don't feel the "want," you lose an erection, you don't get an erection, you come too soon, or you don't come at all), it doesn't mean that sex mustn't happen or that it must end. You can still have a pleasurable experience with your partner because pleasure is your value guiding the shared experience.

2. Values Are Freely Chosen

Since your adolescent years, you've been inundated with messages about how you *should* live your life. These messages flooded in from authority figures of all types: parents, schoolteachers, clergy, media, and entertainment. *"Boys must be brave, courageous, confident and certainly not cry or be vulnerable,"* and *"Good girls should be nice, polite, deferential, and accommodating."*

It reminds me of my patient Karen, who shared the following story: *"When I was about 12, I spent the summer with my much older sister. We'd go to the beach nearly every day. One day, my sister said, 'You've got to shave those legs. Your hair is growing in. Don't you want to look pretty, Karen?'"*

Karen, of course, didn't realize that she was being domesticated to equate shaved legs with beauty. And since beauty resides "in the eye of the beholder," Karen was then and still is now shaving her legs so that others would see her as attractive.

Another patient, Dante, grew up in a predominantly male-oriented culture. He'd listen to how other men and boys talked about sex. Moreover, he'd notice how some would face ridicule for mishaps made in learning the art of dating and sex with digging comments such as, *"Do you even know how to eat pussy?"* and *"You better not come too soon—she'll leave your ass!"*

These and similar remarks made for a complicated coming of age. Dante was domesticated to believe that men should know everything about sex and sexuality, despite having little to no access to quality sex education. Worse, he wouldn't be caught dead by his friends with books on the topic for fear that it would confirm with them that he doesn't know shit! (Odds are this might be the first non-fiction book that you've read about sex and sexuality!)

Karen and Dante adopted beliefs that reflected values held by others; they didn't freely choose them themselves. Values are not the unwanted, passive byproducts of one's childhood domestication. The genuine nature of values mirror what's important to you when you self-reflect. They should be inspirational and provide an emotional lift when you think about them and how well they represent the authentic *you*.

How can you differentiate between freely chosen values and those forced upon you? Here's a clue: echoes of domestication are heard when your mind-chatter includes concerns and worries such as *"I must,"* *"I should,"* and *"I have to."*

Opposite of that, evidence of your values is heard when your self-reflections of the person you want to be include encouraging statements such as *"I get to,"* *"I choose to,"* and, *"I want to."* Notice how the former feel heavy while the latter feel light. The latter statements reflect inspiration while the former reflect subjugation.

3. Values Are Not Emotions

It's easy to confuse emotions with values. Feelings are temporary whereas values are more enduring. For example, one of the most common reasons clients cite for coming to therapy is "to be happy." Being happy sounds like a value, but it's a feeling—and a temporary one at that. Values are permanent whereas permanent feelings would be maladaptive. All a feeling does is reflect your current relationship with your environment. Feelings provide feedback about whether the environment—be it what's occurring in your head or outside of your head—is comfortable or uncomfortable.

On the other hand, a value demonstrates what's important to you, and your pursuit of what's important helps create a context that promotes a particular feeling, such as happiness.

When couples see me and one partner states an emotion as a value, such as a need to feel more desired by the other, I ask them these kinds of questions: *"What is it about feeling desired that's important to you? How is it communicated to you? How would your partner know that you are feeling more desired?"*

This introspective inquiry elevates the conversation away from criticism and blame and more toward greater understanding, compassion, and empathy. This self-reflection helps your partner to reason, *"Oh, okay, that makes sense to me now."* Discussions about values help provide a needed context at times to disarm a feeling or emotion, enabling you to getting more of what you want. For example, you and your partner provide this context when you choose and name your love rocks, your values through which passion can thrive.

4. Values Are Not Wants or Needs

The problem for us OCs is that getting our wants, needs, and expectations met by our partners is totally out of our control. You can ask your partner to meet a need or fulfill a request, but it's ultimately up to them whether they'll do what you ask them to do.

An example of treating a value as a need is your valuing honesty, but your need for honesty is conditional upon your partner never lying. You're misleading yourself then because you can't control whether your partner will tell the truth or lie. Your partner's lying is not a violation of your value of honesty; _your_ lying is a violation of your value of honesty. You don't want to impose your values on others, but do you want to stay with someone who disagrees with your values? It's a choice that you make. This goes back to the precept that values are freely chosen.

When we're talking about needs, we often confuse them with the concept of preferences. The reality is, if you don't have something, you mustn't need it. Unfortunately, many OCs perceive an inability or unwillingness to meet a need or fulfill a request as evidence that the other doesn't love them. It's as if there's an embedded rule, *"If you loved me, you would do this. In fact, if you REALLY loved me, I wouldn't even have to ask you; you SHOULD just know."*

For example, Shantelle and Ben came to see me regarding relationship distress, which included a history of infidelity. During a session, Shantelle said that she found a broken cock ring in a bag on their bedroom floor. She recognized it as a cock ring that she and Ben had used together, but she had no context for why it was broken. She and her partner didn't break it. Therefore, based on their history of infidelity, she assumed that her partner broke it while cheating on her.

Naturally, her thought was, *"I need to know the truth."*

Okay. Now hold yourself, because the shit's going to get real here. Are you ready?

Shantelle doesn't *need* to know the truth in the sense of not surviving without knowing the truth. It was her preference to know the truth. How do I know? Because she was alive in that moment without knowing the truth. In other words, she mustn't have needed to know the truth because she was existing without it. If you don't have it, you mustn't need it.

Here's another example. Becky is a high-level executive at a pharmaceutical company and is intensely overcontrolled. She lost her shit when she discovered bills that her wife had misplaced that were now past due. As an OC person, Becky has this rule: *"I never miss a payment. In fact, I always pay early."*

You can imagine that finding past due bills addressed to her with "Past Due" stamped on the envelope created a cascade of anxiety in Becky. If her credit score dropped because of her partner's irresponsibility, she'd risk feeling embarrassed and humiliated; the event reflected a loss of control of her detail-focused, perfect world. The thought of her score being lower than that of her family and friends was too much for her to bear; she just couldn't live with that comparison.

Now, OCs typically have a high degree of self-control, but when they're pushed to the brink, they can experience "emotional leakage," a term describing OCs when they drop the veneer that *"everything is fine."* Becky's growing frustration with her wife's irresponsibility lit a fuse. Becky persistently tried various strategies to put the fuse out, but she couldn't resolve her resentment with her wife's behavior. And as with any lit fuse, it eventually ignites the gunpowder, and BOOM!

We call this emotional leakage because OCs pride themselves on their ability to stay calm during most situations. Becky's ego reached its tipping point, and in her emotional outburst, she told her partner that she had to leave. Staying with such an irresponsible and inconsiderate person would violate Becky's value of integrity. She'd rather be alone than to live with the "inconveniences" of accommodating another's way of being in the world. Sound familiar?

During my therapy with Becky, I got her to realize that she believed that a rule had been broken, which fueled her emotional leakage. She was treating her value of integrity as if it were a goal or a rule fueled by fear. *"I have to pay my bills on time because I would never want anybody to think that I was less than responsible."*

The question is, are you willing to live with a partner who doesn't mirror your values perfectly? Would it violate your value of integrity, for example, to stay with your partner given whatever it is they're doing that rubs you the wrong way? Your ego has a way of redefining preferences as needs, which fuels a sense of urgency, making you vulnerable to feeling neglected, abandoned, disrespected, et cetera.

If, however, you override that mind chatter and define your needs as preferences, they immediately feel lighter. A need is a requirement; a preference is not. You would love to have it—as Becky would love to have demonstrations of responsibility out of her wife—but you're capable of staying psychologically flexible in the moment if you don't get it.

Psychological flexibility allows you to adapt and remain close to your values while honoring the other's ability to live by their set of values. OCs can become so rigidly attached to an outcome that it deprives them of the ability to accommodate the moment.

Whereas outcomes aren't always in your control, values are always within your direct control. Your values don't represent how *your partner should be* but rather the kind of partner *you want to be*. In making nice with naughty, this includes showing up as the sexual and relationship-oriented being that you are. Values are always about self, the ideal self. However, this isn't about perfection. Perfection is a standard born out of anxiety and worry associated with the fear of not being perfect.

5. Values Are Not Conditional

In the context of sexual and intimate relationships, values are not conditional or dependent on a particular outcome or upon someone else's behavior. They are all about you and your behavior. It's about your process of getting closer to the kind of person you want to be and the unencumbered sexual being you want to be for your partner.

Returning to the story of Steve and Terry, Terry has a value of being adventurous, and Steve doesn't, and Terry takes a step toward that value by making an exciting request of Steve. But Terry doesn't get the outcome that he hoped for. Steve's body responds by tightening up and becoming rigid out of fear. He feels anxious inside, which leads him to become angry and agitated with himself and the situation Terry put him in, which causes Steve to emotionally and physically push Terry away. Terry, in turn, gets mad at Steve for assuming that his adventurous moves would ever be meant to put Steve in harm's way.

Steve is engaged in this process of what's called "experiential avoidance." Nearly everyone engages in one form of experiential avoidance or another. Essentially, this avoidance occurs whenever you're unwilling to be with uncomfortable internal experiences (thoughts, memories, feelings, sensations) while also pursuing ways to avoid or control those uncomfortable experiences. Steve's intrusive thoughts about possible sexual unresponsiveness will cause him to feel uncomfortable and anxious, so he acts in ways designed to avoid the discomfort such as pushing Terry away. However, those actions don't reflect his values and move him closer toward how he wants to be in the relationship, which is to feel close to Terry.

Should Steve realize that he could bring anxiety along with him toward his values, he would have more of what he ultimately wants, while acknowledging Terry for what he wants. For example, when Terry comes up from behind Steve and hugs him, Steve can lean back into the anxiety even more by grabbing Terry's arms and wrapping them more tightly around him, even though his mind chatter is telling him to freeze. Steve can choose to tell anxiety *"I'm the boss here"* and receive the moment.

When I talk to couples about their patterns of relating to each other, the questions I typically ask are often quite revealing for them: *"How workable is it for you to respond as you do when your partner shares a desire or concern? Is that moving your relationship in the direction you want to go? Are you feeling closer toward those things that you say are important to you for you and your partner to share?"*

Ask yourself, when you're with your partner, are your rationalizations, emotions, and resulting behaviors moving your relationship in the direction you want it to go? When it comes right down to it, there are only one of two ways to engage with your partner:

with a closed heart, or with an open heart. When you're living out your values, your heart is open and willing. You'll have clarity and direction on who you want to be as a sexual person and will more often choose sexual and intimate behaviors that reflect your values.

6. Values Are Not Deficits

Values representing your personal beliefs about what's important to you. They guide you in your attempts to live an authentic life as an unfettered and confident sexual being. The challenge for OCs though is that we love to use values as metrics for assessing and comparing what others lack or need to improve on. When this occurs with one's partner, it has the effect of making the partner appear less desirable. In short, their perceived flaws become magnified, which decreases attraction.

Values, therefore, are not to be used as tools to label weaknesses or deficits in yourself or identify failings or shortcomings in others. Instead, values clarify what's important to you so that you can set your sights on moving toward what matters most in your life. Even if you act consistently in your values, it still helps to identify them. Defining them and setting them out as your guideposts encourages you to be mindful of your actions and assess and continuously calibrate your behaviors with your values—with your North Star.

7. Values Rarely Conflict

There will be times when you feel your values conflict with one another. Sam, for instance, was domesticated to believe that she had to be great at everything—family, career, sports—consequently, she carries tons of anxiety on her shoulders about showing up imperfectly. She becomes hypervigilant and thinks about her children while at work, constantly checking the daycare center's nanny cam. When at home, she ruminates about work, constantly checking her email. If you're a woman in our culture, particularly a woman, you've been programmed to believe that you can have it all if you only worked hard enough.

Consequently, for OCs, "having it all" has become synonymous with being dutiful in living life right.

Men can receive similar messages from their mind chatter, but they're often much more limited. Men as boys are told that they must be dutiful at their careers and provide, which usually comes at the expense of the needs of a young family. And, with young children and a spouse at home, the cost of such neglect can be high, not to mention isolating.

It's easy to assume that you're experiencing a values conflict when frustration surfaces from competing demands. A common misperception is that there must be a values conflict between career and family if there's tension between these two domains of your life. However, values conflicts are relatively rare. In this instance of career versus family, the conflict isn't regarding what's important; the conflict arises because there is either a time conflict, a rules conflict, or both.

A time conflict can be recognized easily if you answer yes to the following: *"If I had all of the time in the world, would I devote time to everything important to me?"* If yes, then it's not about a conflict between career and family, or work and leisure. Rather, it's a *time* conflict where you do not have sufficient time to devote to all that's important to you.

More often, though, we OCs find ourselves having rules conflicts. Rules conflicts occur when we've internalized ways of being in the world, which usually comes in the form of the *shoulds, musts,* and *have tos* that get in the way of focusing our thoughts and energy on more meaningful activities and relationships.

Here's an example. Tony was scared. He hadn't had sex with Megan before marrying her five years ago. They remained celibate until marriage to please God. Once married, they had sex a few times, but Megan developed a chronic health condition that made sex feel painful at times. Tony adored his wife and was committed not to cause her pain. He wanted a better sex life with her but was paralyzed by the idea of trying something different. He believed that the only proper sex was missionary style. On the other hand, his wife grew tired of the same old, same old. Yet, missionary was all Tony knew; it was familiar, safe, and comfortable. He liked vanilla sex; it got the job done. It was reliable, and it worked for him.

Given his limited knowledge and exposure to sexual information, Tony felt anxious about the thought of trying something different from what he had experienced before. He shuddered at the thought of feeling awkward or risking embarrassment if something went wrong. He told himself that trying something different, like introducing sex toys into the bedroom, violated his morals or how sex *should* be.

You see, Tony thinks he's experiencing a values conflict, but, as mentioned, values conflicts are relatively rare. Instead, he's experiencing a rules conflict between what constitutes "healthy sex" and his unconscious rules such as, *"I must decide for my wife about what's tolerable for her instead of having her decide for herself,"* and *"I must remain comfortable and not try new things that might feel awkward; I can't feel awkward."*

The major causes of sexual problems with overcontrolled people are rules conflicts. *"I have to be perfect sexually."* Being a perfect lover becomes a prerequisite, and that perfect sex means freedom from uncomfortable outcomes and their associated feelings. *"Sex must unfold perfectly, where no one gets upset, and everyone orgasms."*

Count the rules in that statement: sex must unfold perfectly, no one should be upset, and perfect sex must include orgasms. Rigid adherence to a set of rules throws cold water on desire. Making nice with naughty is essentially about breaking the rules. It's finding and embracing a level of comfort with discomfort.

EXERCISE: VALUES CHECK

We just spent the last couple of pages discussing a general explanation of what values are and are not; and now that we're on the same page, you can be more discerning in your thinking. You have a clearer explanation of the nature of values in the context of sexual and intimate relationships.

We're now going to use the following questions to help you apply the knowledge you've just been given to help you articulate your values relative to sex and sexuality. If you're honest with your answers, this values check will guide you when you're starting to feel awkward or anxious, worried, and judgmental.

Your answers to the following questions will help illuminate your values:

1. What kind of sexual partner do you want to be? (For example, do you want to be a sexual partner who is present, engaged, invested, accepting, curious, playful?)

1. What's vital for you in having a satisfying and fulfilling sexual relationship?

2. What kind of sexual partner do you want to be when your OC temperament gets the best of you?

3. Think of people whose sexuality you admire. What are they doing that captures your attention? You're not judging them; you're being open. You're looking for what you think is inspiring them from within.

4. What kind of sexual partner do you want to be when you feel awkward, insecure, or impatient? Reflect on what the opposite of withdrawal would be in order to stay present and in the moment with your partner? What would your behavior be so you would be sending messages that are more pro-relational than anti-relational?

5. What kind of sexual partner do you want to be when you aren't feeling the "want" to have sex, but your partner is interested? Do you want to be a *"yes and"* partner or a *"no"* partner? What would your behavior be so you would be sending messages that are more pro-relational than anti-relational?

Choosing Naughty Actions

Often, being naughty isn't a reflection of sexual behavior. Being naughty can mean rebelling against old, worn-out sexual scripts about what being a sexual person is, how a sexual person thinks, and how a sexual person behaves. Being naughty can also mean rebelling against expectations and rules thrust upon you by authority figures and society. Moreover, being naughty can mean you are acting in ways contrary to past behaviors so that you're getting more of what you want.

Now that you have a handle on what's important to you relative to how you want to show up as a sexual person, it's time to use your values as guideposts. Keep in mind that your values are not destinations but are helpful guides for navigating through life by opening your heart and choosing behaviors that move you closer to what you want and closer to your partner. Making nice with naughty requires changing how you think (cognitions) and what you do (behaviors), even when emotional obstacles might distract you from what's important.

Let's put it to the test. Let's bring your values to life by exploring and clarifying the actions that reflect your values in the context of your sexuality and intimacy. We'll then unearth the obstacles of your thoughts and feelings that could get in the way of your making nice with naughty.

EXERCISE: VALUES CLARIFICATION

In this exercise, I would like you and your partner to explore each of the words you used to build your love fire together at the end of Chapter 5. Those words are the safe, sane, and consensual values that allow you to express your passion for each other. But before that, let's broaden the language to include all aspects of values that may be anxiety provoking. Here are examples of values found in Lev and McKay's book that might be important to you as a sexual person.[26] Feel free to add additional values in the blanks provided.

Accepting	Cleanliness	Authenticity
Adventurous	Honesty	Laughter
Appreciative	Loyalty	Compassion
Assertive	Trust	Growth
Attentive	Respect	Connection
Attuned	Communication	Security
Available	Forgiveness	Reassurance
Committed	Vulnerability	Empathy
Attractiveness	Companionship	Reciprocity
Openness	Empowerment	Admiration
Understanding	Spirituality	Awareness
Engagement	Creativity	Kindness
Loving	Sensuality	Spontaneous
Dependable	Trustworthy	Mindful
Courage	Willingness	

Now, combine the words on your love rocks with your choices from the list above. You can also add values from other areas of your life. You'll find that you've accumulated many values through this process, so your next step will be to reduce that list to the 10 most important values you and your partner share. Granted, it's a challenge for us OCs to whittle down a list. We tend to think everything is

---

[26] Lev & McKay (n 25), p 54.

important and that everything is *equally* important. It can't be that way for this exercise though, so you'll have to reduce your number of values down to those 10 that you consider as your core values.

Your last prioritization now is to take your list of 10 and order them from most to least important and complete the following table by describing in column three the naughty actions you would take.

Let's say for this exercise that your number one value in a sexual and intimate relationship is being "spontaneous." What behavior would you exhibit as a reflection of being spontaneous in this example? What are the thoughts that you might have about being spontaneous? What does spontaneity mean to you? What actions in your mind inspire spontaneity?

Here are some thought starters for you. Continue this exercise by listing each of your 10 core values and the inspired actions you would be presenting to your partner as a reflection of those values.

Value	Naughty Action
Spontaneity	When I'm feeling horny, I immediately tell my partner. I text naughty thoughts to my partner whenever I have them, even if I'm having lunch with my friends at work.

Now that you have identified your values and the actions that you'll be taking, it's essential to consider what obstacles might be present that could get in the way of your making nice with naughty. For each of the 10 core values, reflect on those thought- and feeling-obstacles blocking your actions.

Value	Naughty Behavior	Thoughts that might get in the way	Feelings that might get in the way	Putting naughty into action, when will you take action?	Are you willing to feel these thoughts and feelings and still take action?
Spontaneity	Text naughty thoughts.	Someone else seeing the text. Feeling embarrassed.	Anxiety over being exposed. Fear of being rebuffed.	When I accept that it's natural to feel awkward when trying new things.	Yes

You have years of domestication that have led to the development of your particular set of obstacles. In addition, as an OC, you have a biotemperament that has features that can also present themselves as obstacles, such as your need for perfection and safety. In other words, obstacles are expected. However, their presence doesn't necessarily call for your paralysis.

The purpose of identifying and describing your values is to illuminate a path forward for yourself and your partner. It's to help you think through how you want to be sexual and intimate with each other and what specific changes you're willing to make to in order to continuously move toward each other using your values as guideposts.

In the next chapter, your journey will be made lighter as you learn how to imaginatively, emotionally, and physically practice thinking and acting differently. You'll develop specific strategies for demystifying the anxieties that are blocking your progress toward what you truly want as a sexual being and how you authentically want to show up in the world.

You'll learn how to change your relationship with anxiety and shift from expending your energy in treating anxiety as an enemy to gathering strength from it by embracing it as a friend. You could bring anxiety along with you, out of the desert and toward your values, and ultimately have more of what you want—expressing and finding enjoyment in your sexuality.

CHAPTER 7

MAKING FRIENDS WITH ANXIETY

"When you change the way you look at things, the things you look at change."

— Dr. Wayne Dyer

Sally is no stranger to anxiety. Much of her life emphasized managing worries and apprehensions. She cultivated an environment where life felt predictable and outcomes felt certain. Sally grew up in a religiously conservative community in Utah. While she didn't practice the predominant faith, she was immersed in the beliefs of the church community, which regarded premarital sex and masturbation as sins against God, and that sex outside of marriage made one impure. Throughout Sally's early life, there was a heavy emphasis on controlling "impure" thoughts, dressing modestly, and being demure in her behavior. Sex, consequently, took on a tone of fear, trepidation, and paranoia.

Subsequently, Sally met Jeremy at the local university where they worked. Both were recruited to collaborate on a committee and began to spend considerable time together. Sally was particularly drawn to Jeremy's laid-back West Coast upbringing. The values and beliefs that Jeremy and his family held were particularly appealing to Sally. His family seemed so carefree, loving, and accepting compared to the norms and mores of her childhood.

Sally and Jeremy dated for six months and decided to wait until they were married to have sex. But even though they are married now, Sally's fear and anxiety about the act of sex, even thinking about it, have contributed to a number of problems, including dyspareunia (painful intercourse) whenever she's intimate with Jeremy. Note that the causes of dyspareunia can be varied and include both physical and psychological factors. Sally's symptoms resulted from the emotional burden of sexual shame she acquired over the course of her life. And although Sally loves Jeremy, she couldn't shake off the effects of her childhood domestication. Sex and anxiety became wedded to one another. She struggled with divorcing the two (i.e., sex and anxiety) so she and Jeremy could experience sexual pleasure and fulfillment.

A stern religious background and rigid beliefs can cultivate unhealthy levels of anxiety across various human experiences. These beliefs may impede the development of a flexible attitude that enables making nice with naughty possible. Often with good intentions, parents inadvertently impose this anxiety onto their children, particularly their daughters. When it comes to sex, societal norms and expectations tend to be more restrictive and rules-based for females than for males. Parents fear the shame, embarrassment, and humiliation that could occur if their daughters become pregnant. Consider the social concept of virginity; it's been synonymous with the notion of purity for thousands of years, and for millennia mostly concerned females. No one ever asks if a guy is a virgin. Well, not often.

Besides religion, many OCs' anxieties related to sex are a product of sexual perfectionism and the perceived rules associated with sex. OCs are vulnerable to imposing restrictive rules on themselves, their partners, and their environment (i.e., in how specific environmental conditions must be met). The assumption with these rules is that they provide needed levels of safety and security for sex to be enjoyable. However, rarely are conditions "good enough"; there are always more perfect conditions to be had. The negative fallout from these beliefs isn't limited to the one who holds them; there's collateral damage, too. Partners who feel under the microscope of hyper-perfectionism can develop sexual insecurities as well, which may lead to arousal issues such as low libido, erectile disappointment, or difficulty lubricating.

My intent in this chapter is to help you change your relationship with anxiety, learn to live with it, and even draw strength from it to reclaim your innate sexual self. I intend to facilitate your making friends with your fears, worries, and concerns by helping you distinguish healthy from unhealthy forms of anxiety and separate rational from irrational thoughts. You'll learn strategies to support your new reasoning by disputing irrational beliefs and will experience the positive effect healthier thoughts can have on your sex life.

Yes, I'm asking you to change your relationship with your anxiety and benefit from its presence. What do I mean by benefit? Consider this parallel: the Yerkes-Dodson Law is a principle based on an observable relationship between stress (anxiety) and performance. The law states that performance increases with stress, but only up to a point. When the level of stress becomes too high, performance decreases.[27] Thus, an optimal level of stress corresponds to an optimal level of performance. Another way to look at it is that stress, to a point, doesn't negatively affect performance but enhances it.

Likewise, there are degrees of anxiety and a similar relationship between anxiety and sexual performance where an optimal level of anxiety (stress) corresponds to an optimal level of sexual performance. You can achieve that optimum balance for you by learning to live with your anxiety, find that point of open co-existence, and put it to work for you in your sexual and intimate relationships.

---

[27] Nickerson, Charlotte (November 15, 2021). *The Yerkes-Dodson Law and Performance.* Simply Psychology. Retrieved from https://www.simplypsychology.org/what-is-the-yerkes-dodson-law.html

Confronting Your Anxiety-Producing Beliefs

The very first step in finding that ideal balance in your consciousness is to observe your mind's production of thought. Contrary to what many self-help books report, you *cannot control* what thoughts arise or when they surface. Moreover, you can't rid yourself of thoughts. (Try *not* to think of a banana. What just happened? Banana, right?) Instead, you *can change* your relationship with the thoughts your mind produces.

Let's use an example to which many OCs can relate—wanting to be "good at sex." This thought fuels the pressure to perform sexually and intensifies the worry of not meeting your—or your partner's (assumed)—expectations. You're afraid that you'll make a fool out of yourself and feel embarrassed and ashamed by your self-perceived inadequacies. Naturally, your sympathetic nervous system gets activated, and you begin to feel anxious. The mind floods with chatter about sexual "musts" and "have tos" such as:

"I must show up perfectly as a sexual partner; nothing unexpected must happen."

"I must mind read and know exactly what to do and when to do it."

These rules raise the stakes and lower your confidence. Consequently, you're consumed with more thoughts of failing and being rejected by your partner, which causes you to feel even more anxious. As Yerkes-Dodson Law would predict, too much anxiety diminishes your ability to show up sexually.

In case it isn't apparent, anxiety in this instance is *not* an aphrodisiac; it doesn't enhance your sexual performance. Your intense alertness to your fears consumes both your thoughts and all your sexual energy. You may not even be attuned to what your body is feeling or what you're communicating to your partner. Your mind chatter becomes a worry machine, churning out worry after worry after worry. You might even experience physiological responses such as body shakes, stomach issues, and muscle paralysis.

In any anxiety-producing situation, you have parts that you have control over and parts that you have no control over. This Dichotomy of Control is one of the underlying tenants of Stoicism, a philosophy of life (that I'll share more on shortly) that strengthens positive emotions and lessens negative ones by separating things that are within our control, our thoughts and actions, and things that are outside of our control, literally everything else.

The Serenity Prayer, made well known by Alcoholics Anonymous, offers a similar message that reads: *"God grant me the serenity to accept the things I cannot change, the courage to change the things I can, and the wisdom to know the difference."*

Focusing on those things we cannot control happens to be a great source of anxiety for us OCs. When it comes to making nice with naughty, I encourage you to focus on what you can control or influence, such as your beliefs, specifically cultivating rational beliefs that reflect what you would like to have happen. The next time you feel sexually anxious, consider maintaining the following rational thought instead:

I would love to have a good time with my partner. I would love to feel desire, have my body respond as I wish, and please both myself and my partner.

I may not feel desire or experience my body responding in ways I would prefer, which would be unfortunate. I won't get what I want, and my partner might be disappointed or upset. However, having a body that doesn't respond according to my preferences and having a sexually frustrated partner won't be the end of the world. It may be disappointing and inconvenient, but it isn't the end of the world.

If there's any hope of turning your OC dial down on your anxieties, it will come from connecting with the real *you* behind all of that worry. Remember, y*ou* are not your experience; *you* are that one who observes your experience. *You* are not anxious; instead, *you* are the awareness of the feeling of anxiety inside of you. You can think your way through to being more flexible in your sexual behaviors and pursuing alternatives that are still pleasurable for you and your partner. Even if your sexual problems persist, you might experience personal disappointment, but *you* won't be destroyed.

If your preferences continue not to be realized, you'll endure and show up as an open and willing sexual partner. You'll do the best with what you've got because you want your partner to experience your desire to feel close to them and attend to their sexual needs.

The Different Forms of Anxiety

Anxieties differ from normal feelings of nervousness or anxiousness and often involve excessive fears or concerns, usually over an impending or anticipated event or outcome. For some, in the context of intimate relationships, it can come in the form of worrisome thoughts about one's subsequent sexual encounter. For others, anxiety is more of a physical sensation such as butterflies in the stomach or irritability. It could also manifest as muscle tension, as Sally experienced in the story above.

Regardless of what form it takes, anxiety has been a mainstay of the human condition and, for that reason, likely contributed to our success as a species. The point is, at its highest level of distinction, there are healthy forms of anxiety.

Healthy Anxieties: Your Friends

Our tendency for cautiousness has been shaped over hundreds of thousands of years of evolution, putting us on high alert when something seems wrong. The ensuing anxiety is experienced, in part, because our bodies release adrenaline and cortisol as part of the sympathetic response. These hormones serve many functions, including preparing us for flight or fight and regulating our stress response.

Anxiety isn't your enemy despite what you've been told by a society and a mental health industry that medicalizes and monetizes distress with "a pill for every ill." I know, I know. It sure feels like an enemy, given how uncomfortable fear and worry can be. However, hear me out. If anxiety was entirely bad and utterly unproductive, natural selection would have evolved that feeling right out of us. Instead, anxiety has remained our constant companion. Anxiety stuck around, and it's here to stay. Why? Because anxiety is your evolutionary friend. It focuses your attention on immediate threats and motivates you to act in ways to preserve the things you want and avoid the things you don't.

Of course, anxiety doesn't feel like a friend when you're experiencing it, but neither does a fever. Yet fevers do good things for your body as well. Fever is not an illness; it's a symptom, or sign, that your body is fighting a disease or infection. It raises your body's temperature to fight off the infection and tells your immune system to make more white blood cells and join in the battle. Similarly, anxiety is simply a warning sign that focuses your attention on a real or imagined threat.

However, like some friends and family members, anxiety can overstay its welcome and transmute into unhealthy thoughts and emotions. At that point, the anxiety becomes maladaptive, leading to a host of psychological, physical, and interpersonal problems, especially when the object of the anxiety is misperceived and misinterpreted.

Unhealthy Anxieties: Your Unfounded Fears

Here's the deal: your mind does a shitty job differentiating between your thoughts and reality. When reality hits and danger is present, your body responds either with flight, fight, or freeze. Similarly, when you get sucked into the mind-chatter of the ego, your body responds to those thoughts as if they are real (ergo, the release of cortisol and adrenaline). In other words, your body responds to imagined threats with the same level of hypervigilance as if they were real threats. In essence, you feel what you think. Let me share an example of what I mean.

Like so many people, Megan believes that she must have the feeling of "want" to have sex with Kirstie. However, she hardly ever feels the "want" and feels terrible about it, contributing to their problems. Add to that, Megan also feels anxious whenever Kirstie pursues her sexually without a clear sense of mutual desire on Megan's part. In those moments, Megan would internally ask herself, *"Do I want to have sex?"* and sensing no desire, rejects Kirstie's advances.

Consequently, Megan's mind begins projecting into the future where she encounters another incident with Kirstie where she doesn't register desire for her impromptu advances. Megan imagines the look of disappointment washing across Kirstie's face again. In other words, Megan experiences *anticipatory anxiety*—anxiety about experiencing anxiety in the future.

Megan's anxiety is a product of irrational thinking. The truth is that most unhealthy forms of anxiety are products of various irrational thought processes such as exaggeration, oversimplification, overgeneralization, unexamined illogical assumptions, faulty deductions, absolutistic ideas, and demands that emotions, thoughts, or realities do or do not exist.

When you're confronted with unhealthy forms of anxiety that get in the way of making nice with naughty, the best course of action is to, again, focus on what you have control over—your thought process. However, like many OCs, you may start wondering, *"Why should I change my thinking? It's helped me to get where I am today. It's been an effective way to live my life. Besides, if I change my way of thinking, wouldn't that mean I would exert less control, which is the opposite of what I want. I want more control, not less. With more control, I'd be less anxious about sex and relationships."*

Wow! Okay. That was a lot of mind-chatter there! Let's slow it down.

I suspect your strategies for confronting anxiety aren't as effective in the sexual and relationship domains of your life. Those strategies may work wonders in your work life and collegial or distant relationships, but your intimate relationship and sex life are suffering under that line of reasoning. Indeed, if your strategies work, continue with them. However, if those strategies aren't getting more of what you want, adopt new approaches and acquire new skills. Start taming the inner-critic and negative mind-chatter that routinely holds you back from the intimacy that awaits you.

Rational and Irrational Beliefs

Most OCs within my practice pride themselves on thinking rationally and often exalt their use of logic. They experience great admiration for their ability to think through various scenarios and devise solutions that mitigate problems for themselves and others. This is why employers love OCs on their teams; they solve problems and get shit done.

Many OCs trust every thought their mind produces—in essence, they become compulsive buyers of their mind-chatter and then pride themselves on thinking rationally. In actuality, their propensity for rational thinking and their advice are often products of an ego that whips up irrational thoughts to exert more control over a situation. In short, OCs can inflate their rational ability by emphasizing incidences of positive outcomes and ignoring the many times when worry and hypervigilance proved useless.

Because you appear to others as having your life together, I suspect you often find others coming to you for advice. Even if they don't ask for it, OCs will offer unsolicited advice when clear solutions are apparent. Sometimes this "accept my advice, fix the problem so we can move on" approach can be the source of much consternation within relationships! Sound familiar?

In building on the skills that I've covered in previous chapters, we're going to look at methods for addressing anxiety-producing beliefs and employing rational beliefs that move you closer to what you want—expressing and finding enjoyment in your sexuality and increasing sexual desire and intimacy between you and your partner.

Rational Emotive Behavior Therapy

As I shared earlier in Chapter Three, Dr. Albert Ellis, in 1955, pioneered a straight-talk approach to psychotherapy called Rational Emotive Behavior Therapy (REBT).[28] Ellis found that classical psychoanalysis, with its incessant focus on early childhood experiences, didn't lead to the behavioral change people wanted. Fundamentally, and drawing from the Stoics (a school of philosophy that teaches the development of self-control and courage to overcome destructive emotions),[29] Ellis believed feelings and suffering are primarily influenced by how we think.

Therefore, people change by changing how they think about their lives and taking actions that move them in the direction they want to go and to live the life they want to live. Thus, REBT has its roots in supporting people to engage in life adaptively through teaching specific skills such as assertiveness, social engagement, and conflict resolution, as well as refuting and replacing cognitive errors such as anxiety and depression that entrench people in their emotional problems.

Dr. Ellis's experience in helping his patients realize the root cause of their suffering is what I explore with my patients today. I often discover that the primary cause of patients' anxieties in their sexual and

---

[28] The Albert Ellis Institute. *About Albert Ellis, Ph.D.* Retrieved from https://albertellis.org/about-albert-ellis-phd/.

[29] Stanford Encyclopedia of Philosophy (April 10, 2018). *Stoicism.* Retrieved from https://plato.stanford.edu/entries/stoicism/.

intimate relationships is rarely the situation but their thoughts about it, specifically how they evaluate it. Their inner critic—the embodiment of their ego—narrates their lives in these instances, prods them to accept as fact thoughts that aren't true, and prevents them realizing sexual enjoyment and fulfillment.

REBT lends itself as a practical method to help patients identify irrational beliefs—the root of their anxieties—and better manage their thoughts, emotions, and behaviors in a healthier, more realistic way. To help facilitate that process, Ellis established the ABC model as a core component of REBT, what he terms the ABCs of emotional disturbance: the **A**ctivating event, when a perceived threat happens in the environment around you, triggering your negative emotional or behavioral response; your core **B**eliefs, which describe your thoughts attached to your response; and the **C**onsequence, which is your actual emotional response and action taken as a result. The basic idea underlying the ABCs is that external events do not cause anxieties but that irrational beliefs do and that we have the power to change those beliefs.

Ellis's ABC model is a significant component of REBT. It teaches people with sexual problems their ABCs of emotional disturbance and helps them acquire the tools to change their beliefs and consequences significantly. Those tools complete Ellis's model by assisting patients to **D**ispute their irrational beliefs and experience the new **E**ffect of healthier beliefs and the healthier consequences resulting from those new beliefs.

What follows are the methods you can use to debunk and deconstruct your negative thoughts and emotions. We'll use Ellis's Rational, Emotive, and Behavioral structure as a guide for these methods to understanding your beliefs, the consequences of your thoughts and actions, and how to dispute your mind chatter to experience a better sex life.

1. Rational: Getting the Information You Lack

Knowledge is a core value for many people. It can free us from our assumptions and biases and help us build better relationships. Knowledge also gives us a greater ability to manage our emotions. REBT reveals a good amount of curative information that patients with sex-related anxiety often lack. This knowledge serves to correct dysfunctional reasonings, such as *"Loving partners are spontaneous when it comes to sex," "Sex mustn't be awkward,"* and *"Loving partners can always and easily get aroused and find satisfaction."*

In this section, I describe two methods—Flexible Fantasies and Anti-Awfulizing/Anti-Absolutizing Strategies—to help OCs achieve an open and flexible attitude toward sex and move them away from their self-defeating, relationship-destroying mind chatter.

Flexible Fantasies

You'll recall from Chapter 3 that OCs experience fixed and fatalistic mindsets when life doesn't unfold for them as planned. Sex just happens to be an area where either of these mindsets can create obstacles to making nice with naughty. Therefore, developing a flexible mindset is most helpful for a shift within your sex life. To that end, REBT uses imaging methods—beneficial for OCs who have difficulty feeling aroused or reaching orgasm—to help you imagine various scenarios and navigate through them openly and adaptably. During these flexible fantasies, you're encouraged to explore your sexuality within the safe comforts of your mind. Here's an example.

Megan struggled with experiencing orgasms with Kirstie. Truth be told, Kirstie is Megan's first female sexual partner. She had several male sexual partners in the past and struggled to experience orgasms with them as well. During those earlier sexual encounters, some of her male partners would pressure Megan into having an orgasm to satisfy their egos. Megan already had a great deal of weight on her shoulders, the heaviest being directing a huge HR department while under the microscope of a domineering boss. Consequently, Megan's work-related stress made her further resent pressures to perform sexually.

When Megan met Kirstie, Megan assumed she wouldn't have to experience that kind of pressure again. And true, while Kirstie never pressed Megan, Megan's prior sexual experiences and perfectionistic tendencies gave way to her incessant inner critic prodding her to prove to Kirstie that she was enjoying sex.

Applying Dr. Ellis's ABC model, Megan's struggle with experiencing an orgasm with Kirstie is the **A**ctivating event, triggering Megan's negative emotional response. The **B**eliefs that command Megan's thoughts, especially those related to perfectionism, are justified (in her mind) because of her prior experiences with male partners and her unfulfilling quest for sexual perfectionism.

As a **C**onsequence, Megan experiences anxiety and struggles to climax for believing she has to fake or rush her orgasms with Kirstie the same way she did for her male partners. In brief, perfectionism and self-imposed high standards are causing the anxiety and sexual withdrawal associated with sexual encounters between Megan and Kirstie. Let's look at a dialogue between Megan and me that occurred during one session.

After reviewing her week and homework, I asked, *"Megan, would you be willing to participate in a mental exercise?"*

"Okay," she responded with a mix of curiosity and uncertainty.

"Nice—you're already showing some flexibility. We're off to a good start. I'd like you to close your eyes, if you will, and imagine being in your most enjoyable, most comfortable place for sex with Kirstie. Let me know when you have this image. Keep in mind that there is no right or wrong way to do this. Whatever you experience is your experience."

"I got the image."

"There you go. Now, imagine that you're engaging in sex with Kirstie despite not having much desire. You're experiencing all of those intrusive thoughts that you normally experience. You're also aware that little is happening in terms of your level of arousal and pleasure. Now, imagine Kirstie showing signs of frustration and irritation that you've not come yet. Imagine Kirstie saying everything you've feared that she would think and say regarding having sex with you. Notice the sensations that arise as you imagine this awful experience. Let me know when you've got this clearly in your mind."

"I've been through this often enough; it doesn't take much effort," Megan half-joked.

"Very good," I said, then asked, "What are the feelings you notice as you imagine this worst-case scenario with Kirstie?"

"Humiliated; inadequate; embarrassed that there's something wrong with me." Megan added, "I'm also angry that I don't experience what seems to come so easily to so many other people."

"I imagine those feelings are very familiar," I acknowledged. "I will now ask that you imagine changing those feelings to only disappointment and frustration. Replace humiliated, embarrassed, and anger with disappointment and frustration."

"That's tough," Megan noted. "The negative thoughts are so intense. It's hard not to feel stronger emotions than just 'disappointment and frustration.'"

"Those thoughts are quite convincing," I added, wanting to make a point of this as the catalyst for a change of thinking. "I'm sure of it, especially when your mind uses you as a tool. In this instance, though, you're using your mind as a tool. In flexible-fantasy, you get to alter your experience. Imagine only feeling frustration and disappointment. Give it a go."

"Okay. I'll give it a try."

"Let me know when there's even the smallest shift toward frustration and disappointment."

Megan took several moments and nodded, indicating a shift.

"Very good. Now, what did you do to make that shift happen?" I asked.

"I suppose I began to talk to myself differently. I recalled some of the things we discussed in therapy about pleasure vs. performance. I reminded myself that I had survived all those other experiences of not having orgasms with my male partners. I also reminded myself that I was able to experience an orgasm at least some of the time. More importantly, I reminded myself that it was my body and my orgasm. There's no rule that I have to orgasm for another person."

"Is there more?" I prompted.

"I told myself that I am not helped by comparing my sexuality to others. Comparing myself to others distracts me from experiencing any pleasure that might arise from having sex with Kirstie. For years I internalized that my orgasms directly impacted my partners' self-worth. They helped me to feel that way, too. Now I realize that it reflected their lack of sexual sophistication and knowledge. My value as a human being isn't tied to my orgasms or the lack thereof," she asserted.

I was delighted with Megan in her ability to articulate her thoughts, and I summarized for her, *"Wow, that's quite impressive and a clearer reflection of reality, Megan. Notice how those thoughts feel different compared to thoughts that you're inadequate or somehow broken. Sure, being disappointed is okay. You aren't getting what you want. Yet, the lack of an orgasm isn't a reflection of your worth or another person's."*

"True. These thoughts feel so much lighter. I remember what you said about lighter thoughts being more closely tied to truth and reality, which makes sense," Megan commented.

"In the coming weeks, I encourage you to engage in flexible fantasy most days of the week. Imagine various stressful scenarios and replace those distressing feelings with mild disappointment and frustration. Then imagine what thoughts supported those feelings. You can see now, however, that your fixed beliefs that you must achieve an orgasm because of their magical ability to determine your and others' worth supported the painful feelings that led to pulling back sexually from Kirstie. Would mild disappointment or frustration be enough to cause you to no longer want sex again, ever?"

Megan chuckled, *"No. It sure wouldn't."*

Several weeks went by before Megan returned for her follow-up appointment. She reported that her flexible fantasy helped her notice when she experienced heavy thoughts. She employed rational beliefs to **D**ispute her irrational beliefs as alternatives that felt lighter and more consistent with reality.

Moreover, Megan found that she could refocus her attention and energy on her body and the pleasure of the moment and experience the new **E**ffect of her healthier beliefs and the improved consequences resulting from those new beliefs. By challenging her old way of thinking, Megan enhanced her ability to feel aroused and experience satisfying orgasms with Kirstie.

Consider using the Flexible Fantasy Exercise at the end of this chapter to help you (1) identify the thoughts your rules-based mind has placed on you (and you may have placed on others) with regards to sexual intimacy; (2) dispute your irrational thoughts; and (3) design a flexible, restorative fantasy of your own.

Anti-Awfulizing and Anti-Absolutizing

The central premise of REBT proposes that people experience problems with their sexuality when they overlay unfortunate past incidents with fatalistic self-beliefs. As a result, they develop absolutistic, perfectionistic expectations of themselves. As you can imagine, anti-awfulizing and anti-absolutizing are important lines of reasoning in REBT therapy.

This cognitive part of the REBT process helps you identify and explore irrational thoughts—your *"I must-haves"*—and actively and insistently challenge and change them to *"It would be better to haves."* These are the different strategies that you can use to practice thinking, feeling, and acting out. After all, if you want something to be different in your life, start with **thinking** and **behaving** differently.

For example, nothing makes it awful (or terrible or horrible) if you cannot achieve a full erection or have an orgasm at what you perceive as "the right time." It may feel frustrating and embarrassing if you don't, but that doesn't equate to it being awful or horrible. "Awful" would be getting third-degree burns over ninety percent of your body. Not getting an erection or becoming lubricated may be inconvenient and disappointing, but there's no benefit to labeling the experience as awful. In short, no matter how inconvenient it is, it never can be more than disappointing and inconvenient.

Look, you may again have sexual experiences that are disappointing; however, being fatalistic about them can trigger thoughts that make you feel even more defective and isolated. The reality is that sexual organs aren't always responsive in the ways we expect. (As I often say to my patients, "Dicks aren't dildos.") Not getting an erection, not having an orgasm, experiencing premature or delayed ejaculation, or having a different level of desire than that of your partner does not make you an imperfect or incomplete person. Shit happens, and when it does, you forge ahead the best you can with what you have available. Nor do you have to be absolutistic about it either by thinking, *"I must never again have this experience happen to me!"* You can still show up as the sexual being you are and satisfy your partner sexually if it does occur.

2. Emotive: Developing Healthy Responses

The best-known aspect of REBT is helping people respond rationally to situations that typically cause stress, anxiety, or depression. This step also includes many emotive-dramatic-evocative exercises for developing healthy responses to situations that I'll outline here.

Shame-Attacking Exercises

How much shame is tied to your struggle to express and find enjoyment in your sexuality? Recall Sally at the opening of this chapter. She believed that her behavior directly impacted her parent's perceptions of themselves as being successful in raising a chaste daughter who was in control of her impure thoughts and desires. The way Sally expressed it, when she didn't make her parents proud, she felt their disappointment profoundly.

OC people tend to score high on conscientiousness, meaning that they are concerned about what other people think about them. This often occurs when one grows up in a family where the parents are vocal about deriving their self-worth from their children's accomplishments or expressing personal vulnerability for their children's failures.

When you have this natural tendency toward overcontrol and then grow up in a family that tends to be very rule-oriented with parents so enmeshed in your life, you can be particularly concerned about your sexual partner's view of you. Because of this rules-based upbringing, Sally's now catching herself doing things that she thinks would disappoint her parents and feeling shame that she's somehow deviant or perverted for having "impure" thoughts. She's put herself into a psychological cage where she's not free to explore her sexuality because of the shame she's feeling.

What is shame but the sense that your personhood is somehow defective. While guilt is, *"I did something bad,"* shame is, *"I am bad."* As you can imagine, shame is incredibly sexually suppressing and interpersonally isolating. You're on guard to avoid situations that might trigger more shame or embarrassment, which stifles the playfulness and spontaneity needed for making nice with naughty.

Overcoming such sexual impediments calls for breaking the chains of shame that have bound you to a history that, in reality, has never served you. One first act of rebellion—a proof point, if you will—is to show up publicly in small ways that might make you appear mildly foolish or ridiculous. You'll discover that your world won't end when you take risks and that others' opinions matter little. As the adage goes, people are far more interested in themselves than you. They're not watching you as attentively or critically as you think.

As you can see from your immediate reaction, this shame-busting exercise of acting silly or looking a little ridiculous in public—even if just for a second—can be challenging for OCs. We expend a lot of energy and effort avoiding the limelight and public displays of even the mildest behavior that would draw disapproval from others.

Being playful is another way of breaking the chains of shame. It's also one of the 14 "Windows of Experience" as defined by father-and-son psychiatrists Thomas and Patrick Malone in their book, *Windows of Experience: Moving Beyond Recovery to Wholeness*.[30] Each "window" is a way of recognizing and developing "our real selves" vis-à-vis the world by changing our old ways of thinking and doing. To "give birth" to yourself, you must, among other windows, accept yourself, accept others, be playful, and take risks.

When you're playful, you're not feeling unhealthy anxiety or stress but relatively healthy anxiousness instead. A sense of well-being and calm comes over you; and for that moment, you're carefree without a worry in the world. Through play, children at a very early age learn to engage and interact with the world around them. They develop social skills and coping skills. They feel safe when they're playing and pretending. It's when they're most happy and naturally expressive.

I always say that the most direct example of play for adults is in their sexuality, where they can safely be childlike, uncomplicated, and naturally expressive. I recently talked about monogamy with a couple who believed that flirting with others outside of the home, even in the mildest and most harmless ways, violates their monogamy contract. It's akin to believing that when they leave their house, they're expected to switch off their sexual nature to avoid getting in trouble for playfully flirting with another person, and then automatically switch it back on as soon as they walk through the front door. Sexuality isn't a toggle

---

[30] Malone, Patrick Thomas & Malone, Thomas Patrick (n 12).

that's flipped on and off at will. You're a sexual being 24/7. These kinds of irrational beliefs about sexuality can fuel sexual repression and act as the lever pressing down on your sexual nature as an individual.

Risk-Taking Exercises

As you may well know by now, OCs are rule-oriented, structured, risk-averse people and hypervigilant to threats that can make them feel vulnerable. As a result, OCs lean toward routine as a source of safety and security. Consequently, they resist taking risks. Risks are often irrationally viewed through a fatalistic lens as horrible and dangerous with uncertain outcomes.

Yet, much like Radically Open Dialectical Behavior Therapy (RO DBT), REBT proposes that routinely engaging in new or different behaviors has the potential to deconstruct old habits, whatever they may be, and help to rewire your brain to where you become okay with engaging in unplanned, risky, spontaneous activities.

As with the shaming exercise above, risk-taking is quite challenging for OCs. This is true even with the smallest kinds of risks. Bill, for example, stopped having sex with Pamela years ago. He loved her, to be sure. He still kissed and hugged her when she came home from work every day. When I asked what their daily reunion ritual was, he said, *"I kiss her three times and hug her. Then we sort of go back to whatever we were doing at that moment."* I encouraged him to kiss her four times and hug her through the awkwardness until he felt relaxed. I wanted him to experiment and observe how changing the routine shifted things even in the tiniest ways.

Another example, perhaps a little riskier, would be asking your partner to engage in a sex act that you fear they would criticize you for. Evolving sexually and personally requires leaning into discomfort via risk-taking so that you can learn new things about yourself and your partner. Taking these minor unpredictable risks that are more focused on pleasure than performance is how you add oxygen and fuel to your fire of desire. You can reaffirm your sexual self by deliberately engaging in naturally expressive imperfect actions to free the playful spirit within you and make nice with naughty.

Emotive Verbalizations

People largely create their emotional anxieties by holding vehemently strong beliefs and negative attitudes about themselves. For example, people struggling to orgasm may feel convinced that they must achieve it and are defective and worthless if unable to orgasm. Imagine how powerfully limiting, distressing, and shame-filled these sentiments are felt within.

You've likely begun your journey with me through this book because you feel that you have a sexual limitation. Perhaps you've come to believe that you have low sexual desire, erectile disappointment, an inability to orgasm, or that you orgasm too quickly. You've undoubtedly fanned the flames of your discontent with yourself with unhelpful statements, such as, *"Isn't it awful or horrible that [fill in the blank] is happening to me?"*

Your mind may have also focused on an element of fairness; for example, *"It's so unfair that I experience this and no one else seems to struggle as I struggle."* Notice how you feel inside amid such statements to yourself. It feels heavy, doesn't it? Now, here's something silly to try. I'd like you now repeat your statement about unfairness, but this time, sing the statement out loud to the tune of "Happy Birthday." Go ahead, I'll wait.

What did you notice about how those very same thoughts feel? Differently, huh? Do you notice how they now feel lighter? From this feeling of lightness, you might reflect on why it would be so awful or horrible if you didn't get as aroused, or you didn't orgasm on cue, and so on. Sure, you might prefer a different experience, but in the end it's not all that terrible. You're still capable of and invited by your partner to engage in other playful forms of connecting.

REBT not only attempts to help you to recognize and call out your anxiety-inducing ideas but to contradict and dispute them in a highly emotional manner. The aim is to gain convincing evidence that you have a right to enjoy and express yourself sexually. To experience this level of freedom, you might have to consider that the rules that have governed your sexual self for all this time may have come from people who held beliefs of you that were never, or will never be, right for you.

3. Behavioral: Acting Your Part

As you've gathered thus far, our rationalizations and emotions are connected. Consequently, an important assumption underlying REBT is that people rarely change and will keep believing strong self-defeating thoughts until they actively take steps to act against those beliefs and emotions and establish anxiety-free muscle memory.

To that end, I encourage my patients to engage behaviorally in sexual activities with themselves (such as masturbation) and with their partners (such as having sex without attempting any intercourse) instead of avoiding those anxiety-producing activities. I encourage couples to work on relationship problems instead of avoiding them and repeatedly practice specific actions until they're proficient at them.

The Big O Reward

REBT employs operant conditioning or self-management techniques, a process by which patients learn to act in such a way as to obtain rewards and avoid punishments. For example, willing patients are taught to reinforce having sex with their partners and penalize (but not berate) themselves when they avoid sex. To that end, my patients and I identify rewards that would encourage them to engage themselves and engage their partners sexually. Let me explain what I mean. Many people have a psychological impediment to masturbating. In one way or another, they've received and still believe messages from their past that masturbation is wrong, sinful, and shameful. Consequently, they've not fully benefited from the sexual self-knowledge that comes with masturbation. In other words, you can better communicate to your partner what you find pleasurable if you've taken the time to discover yourself and what you enjoy.

Additionally, self-management techniques are also used to support the cognitive and emotive changes that I introduced earlier. If willing patients, for example, agree to dispute some of their irrational ideas about how horrible things would be if they failed to get an erection or achieve orgasm, I show them how to reward themselves (and penalize themselves if need be) to increase the probability of their performing their homework assignments.

The Idle Relationship is on a Path to Death

Remember that 1980s infomercial for the Ronco Rotisserie and Barbeque Oven? The advertising slogan was, "Set it and forget it!" Didn't that sound wonderful! You just put the chicken on the rotisserie in the little oven, set the timer, and the appliance does all the rest. Many people do that to their relationship—they set it and forget it—and then it surprises them that the quality of their relationship and fire of desire have diminished due to neglect.

Here's a vivid metaphor to drive home my point: Have you ever driven a car that's out of alignment? If you let go of the steering wheel, the vehicle pulls to the right or left, depending on what side the suspension has failed. Holding on to the wheel to correct and guide your car is analogous to holding on to the wheel of your intimate relationship to keep you and your partner from driving off into a ditch. An idle relationship, one unattended, is most often destined to wither and die. Setting it and forgetting it can never be the path to a vital sexual and intimate relationship.

I know what OCs are thinking right now because I'm tempted to think this way as well: *"If I don't have to introduce anything new and exciting, I don't ever have to fear humiliation, embarrassment, or just being a source of disappointment."*

True, if you do nothing, you won't have to experience those feelings and the anxiety that comes with them. Don't be surprised then when you wake up, peel your forehead off the steering wheel, and find yourself and your car in the ditch. There's only one answer here: never let go of the wheel.

OC folks are highly motivated to rid their lives of discomfort. They see zero value in feeling awkward, embarrassed, or worried. What I'm sharing with you in these chapters are not cures for discomfort. I'm not aiming to help you feel better but rather to help you get better at feeling. Discomfort is not the problem; anxiety is not the problem. Anxiety is simply a feeling that can be disputed to allow new experiences to emerge. Make anxiety your friend by challenging and changing your thoughts, and your behaviors will follow.

CHAPTER 8
TAMING THE MONKEY

"Of course, we can always imagine more perfect conditions, how it should be ideally, how everyone else should behave. But it's not our task to create an ideal. It's our task to see how it is, and to learn from the world as it is. For the awakening of the heart, conditions are always good enough."

— Ajahn Sumedo

Sheri spoke to it plainly as she sat on the couch across from me, *"I can't focus during sex. My mind is flooded with thoughts; it's non-stop. My mind thinks, thinks, thinks. It's so distracting."*

She then recited the compulsive rules and mind chatter that commands her attention and the anxious thoughts that occur whenever she has sex with her partner. She explained how her energy would drop to the point where she couldn't find and enjoy fulfillment in the moment. *"It's either about the laundry that needs to be washed, dishes that are still on the table, the work projects that are piling up, the dress that I need to buy before the weekend. Just non-stop thoughts."* She added, *"Quite frankly, I almost prefer masturbation over sex. When I masturbate, it seems easier for me to enjoy myself. I get to think less about other things. I can focus more."*

Another client experiences distraction differently. Patrick's obstacle to making nice with naughty is his tendency to shut down and become closed-minded whenever his partner wants sex to be spontaneous and playful. As Patrick explains it, *"Her desire for playfulness makes me feel awkward, and I worry about the possibility that I'll embarrass myself or, worse yet, lose my erection."*

His insecurity comes in the form of harsh judgments from his ego. That incessant mind-chatter distracts him from the possibilities and pleasures available to him in the now moment. It compels him to read his partner's invitations as threats to his sense of safety and security.

Patrick's shutting down comes from his feeling of being overwhelmed, one of Thomas Lynch's five classification cues of emotional response that I shared in Chapter 4. While safety, novelty, and rewarding cues are most associated with positive sexuality and intimacy in relationships, threatening and overwhelming cues are our response to stimuli that we've determined to be potentially dangerous or harmful.[31] Moreover, you'll also recall from Chapter 4 that many people experience contextual desire where desire is heavily influenced by environmental factors, which can act as breaks or accelerators. For Patrick, his feeling awkward when his partner is playful slams the breaks on his pursuit of partnered sex.

Granted, being highly sensitive to threatening and overwhelming cues has proved beneficial to OCs in their daily lives. Your sensitivity to these cues gives you a degree of protection similar to having an umbrella when others didn't think to bring one or finding a polyp during an annual physical. Your preparedness in the face of unexpected events can be gratifying, both socially and personally. Unfortunately, being highly sensitive to potential threats in the domain of sexuality and intimacy, which is where many OCs take their uber-preparedness, can cloud your vision and hurt your relationships.

Returning to Patrick, his partner's playfulness becomes too much stimulation. It interrupts his compulsive mental view of how things

---

[31] Lynch (n 1), pp 37–41.

should unfold when engaging in sex in order for him to feel safe and secure. In essence, it triggers fears that he might humiliate or embarrass himself in the future. Because of his partner's mischievousness, the situation that was once under Patrick's control shifts toward more unpredictability, and he becomes overwhelmed with anxiety over the unknown. He shuts down and fatalistically anticipates losing his erection, which causes a cascade of adrenaline that deflates his penis. In short, nothing makes you lose an erection like worrying you'll lose the erection.

Patrick and Sheri, and perhaps you as well, experience mental states where you're preoccupied with memories of the past or anxieties about the future. These thoughts are like virtual reality goggles where you're easily convinced that what the mind sees is actuality. Of course, reality is what you're experiencing in the now moment; everything else is "monkey mind."

Mindfulness Calms the Monkey

When you seriously consider all of the extraordinary moments you've enjoyed over the course of your life, I suspect you would find commonalities in your consciousness: you were fully present, free of distraction and self-criticism, free of wanting the situation to be different, and free of discontent. These qualities also happen to characterize collectively a state of mindfulness. Acclaimed meditation teacher and developer of Mindfulness-Based Stress Reduction, Jon Kabat-Zinn defines mindfulness as the *"awareness that arises through paying attention, on purpose, in the present moment, non-judgmentally…in the service of self-understanding and wisdom."* [32]

---

[32] Mindful Staff (January 11, 2017). *"John Kabat-Zinn: Defining Mindfulness."* Mindful. Retrieved from https://www.mindful.org/jon-kabat-zinn-defining-mindfulness/#:~:text=The%20Definition%20of%20Mindfulness%3A,self%2Dunderstanding%20and%20wisdom.%E2%80%9D

In the absence of mindfulness, you may have noticed your mind acting like a little dancing monkey, jumping up and down, acting erratically and uncontrollably. The monkey's dance moves consist of every mental distraction that keeps you from being present in the now moment. Its antics are quite seductive and hard to keep from noticing. After all, if you're walking down the street and see a dancing monkey, I bet you'll stop, perhaps for a while, and then throw a coin into its owner's hat before moving on. I wouldn't blame you; a dancing monkey is quite captivating. You can see how the Buddhist notion of the monkey mind is evident for Sheri and Patrick in their own individual relationships, each dealing with a mind that produces captivating thoughts that distract them from being in the now moment with their respective partners.

I also bet you have a monkey mind that is all over the place, as evidenced by your painful, stressful, and anxiety-filled relationship with your sexuality. It's this suffering that led you to pick up this book. It may be relieving to know that your suffering doesn't differ all that much from those of your OC compatriots. Your OC mind and my mind are made the same. How is it that I know this? Simple. Besides being similar to dancing monkeys, our egos are like those neighborhoods where every house looks so identical that neighbors accidentally pull into each other's driveway. The lawns are perfectly manicured, the paint combinations are impeccably coordinated, and the picket fences are beaming white.

Though identical on the outside, those houses have very different feels on the inside. Some are compulsively clean and tidy, while others are cluttered and disorderly. Outsiders don't see what's on the inside, and we OCs, in particular, make sure of that. Metaphorically speaking, our shades are always drawn. People assume we have clutter-free minds given our career accomplishments, the appearance of emotional stability, and the Instagram-ready life and family. Moreover, people often admire the homes of OCs; they project steadiness, stability, and maturity. Yet, there's often discontent, uncertainty, and insecurity on the inside. We live alone with our real truths and are intimately (and exhaustedly) aware of the constant stream of monkey-like thoughts that distract us from the present moment. Only you know what it's like to live in your house, to live in your mind. Moreover, only you know how your inner critic can hinder you from getting what you want, especially regarding transformative experiences in your sexual and intimate relationships.

Now that you've accepted who you are and know how your OC temperament affects your capacity to make nice with naughty, this chapter offers a valuable series of meditations designed to help turn down the volume on your mind-chatter. I hope these mindfulness exercises will bring you closer to that optimum balance I mentioned in Chapter 7 by learning to live with your anxiety, making friends with it, and making your mind work for you instead of you working for it.

Mindfulness Meditation for Beginners

Getting started with mindfulness is simple, but don't let its simplicity be confused with ease. The monkey mind that I described above is very entertaining and entrancing. Accordingly, developing greater mindfulness to turn down the chatter requires practice. With the overarching goal in mind of turning down the dial, not off, consider using the following steps to tame your monkey.

First, get seated in a comfortable posture; a proper posture will enhance your focus. I advise that you choose a sitting position over a lying position; otherwise, you might fall asleep. ***Second***, close your eyes or have them three-quarters shut. Some people enjoy staring at something sitting a few feet before them while using a softened gaze. That being said, opened eyes are not ideal for beginners. OC people may become distracted by environmental triggers such as dishes that need to be off the table and in the sink, clothes in the dryer that need to be folded and put away, or floors that needs to be cleaned. ***Third***, bring attention to your breathing: the in-breath, the out-breath. Breath naturally. Alternatively, you might find it useful to employ square-breathing where you inhale for a count of four, hold your breath for a count of four, exhale for a count of four, and inhale again for a count of four. Then repeat the four corners. **Fourth**, when the monkey starts dancing (your mind wanders), accept this as a natural occurrence and simply bring your attention back to your breathing. **Fifth**, do not control anything; just observe.

Self-as-Context

Practicing mindfulness is to live life more fully by being present in an accepting, nonjudgmental way. Mindfulness isn't an easy endeavor, however. Yet as your practice progresses, you'll more easily be able to place space between you and your distressing thoughts, allowing you to express greater values-directed behavior. Separating from your thoughts is a concept we first explored in Chapter 3. Another way of describing this experience is "self-as-context," the perspective from which you observe the content of your thoughts and feelings and how they move in and out of your awareness. It's a place where you're cognizant of your experiences without getting caught up in them. Imagine the relief you would feel if you were free from the grip of your mind-chatter!

Ultimately, freedom is possible because you are not the content of your mind. Instead, you are the observer of your mind. When you observe your mind and question your mind's content, namely the stressful thoughts, your ego lets go of you. There's a feeling of freedom in that moment. By questioning stressful thoughts, you accept the situation for what it is. Through acceptance, suffering diminishes. After all, suffering is pain multiplied by resistance. The more you resist reality, the more suffering you'll experience. Don't take my word for it. Recall your own experiences during times when your suffering was at its greatest, and how acceptance, not resistance or denial, lifted your anguish. This is the essence of mindfulness: that it offers a method for reducing your suffering. Mindfulness is the adaptable, flexible mind that brings attention and awareness to the now moment with openness, patience, and non-judgment. Breathe that in!

Mindfulness makes you slippery to the ego; it's harder for it to grasp you. Your ego losing its hold on you is a distinction that Byron Katie and Stephen Mitchell make in their book, *Loving What Is: Four Questions That Can Change Your Life*. In Chapter 3, I shared Katie's The Work, a method of inquiry designed to ask and listen for answers one finds inside of themselves and open their mind to potentially life-transforming insights. In *Loving What Is*, Katie and Mitchell reason that it's not the problem that causes our suffering; it's our thinking about the problem.[33] Sound familiar? Ellis drew this conclusion in the 1950s, and the Stoics shared this insight more than 2,000 years ago! How's that for longevity?!?

Contrary to conventional wisdom, however, trying to let go of a painful thought without exposing it to the truth never works. Instead, stressful thoughts let go of you once you've questioned the thought and aligned it with reality. At that point, you can truly "love what is" just as it is—freedom.

To reiterate, when you question your mind-chatter, your ego lets go of you. You've become too slippery for the ego to hold onto. When in a state of mindfulness, you're fully in the flow of life, and your ego isn't capable of controlling you and your thoughts. Don't assume your work is done, though. The ego is always looking for an opportunity to become relevant to you once again—to seduce you away from the present moment and smother your peace with mind-chatter. That's

---

[33] Katie, Byron & Mitchell, Stephen (March 19, 2002). *Loving What Is: Four Questions That Can Change Your Life*. p x. Three Rivers Press. Retrieved from, https://www.amazon.com/Loving-What-Four-Questions-Change/dp/0609608746/ref=tmm_hrd_swatch_0?_encoding=UTF8&qid=&sr=

Making Nice with Naughty

why you can come in and out of awareness many times during the course of a day. However, when in a state of mindfulness, you and your mind-chatter are separate, and you are no longer fused with thought.

The Raisin Exercise

Fusion with thought is powerful fuel for suffering, making it difficult and challenging to experience any pleasure, to say the least. Many OCs struggle to find much pleasure from sex because of the distraction of the monkey mind. These distractions may include present experiences (e.g., voices in the hotel hallway) or future concerns (e.g., a work retreat next week). Of course, distractions preventing the experience of pleasure may also be messages from the past (e.g., history of abuse, which we'll cover in Chapter 9, or a parent's assertion that sex is nasty, risky, or sinful). Consequently, OCs are at risk of suppressing their pursuit and experience of sexual pleasure and may need help to acquire greater mindfulness around pleasurable stimulation.

The raisin meditation is a classic mindfulness exercise where you focus on the present moment using all your senses—what you can see, smell, taste, touch and hear—so you can experience pleasure. The idea is that by focusing all your attention on a small fixed object like a raisin, you can clear your mind, bring it into focus, and train your mind to notice the present.

In the context of making nice with naughty, let's use a Hershey's Chocolate Kiss as the object of your attention. Hold the chocolate kiss with your thumb and index finger. Look at it. Notice how the light bounces off the many folds of the tin foil. You might even notice the scent of the chocolate as it travels toward your nose. You feel the wrapper's texture, too: smooth in some areas, not in others. You pull the paper tail (called a *plume*) to open the kiss and inhale the lingering scent of chocolate more deeply.

Now, bring the naked kiss up to your nose. Let it be there for a moment. Notice how the scent of the chocolate has grown more intense. Perhaps you begin to notice nuances to the chocolate that you hadn't seen before. You may notice that your mouth begins to produce more saliva, signaling your body's readiness for pleasure. Allow the anticipation and temptation to build, but instead of popping it into your mouth, just lick it once. Let the flavor wash over your tongue while you continue to breathe in its scent. You may even notice that the heat of your fingers is now melting the chocolate some. Just sit there enjoying those sensations.

Now that you're ready, place the entire chocolate kiss into your mouth and allow it to simply rest on your tongue. No chewing yet. That will come soon. Again, sit there. Observe. Perhaps begin to imagine all the people, plants, animals, et cetera that had a part in this moment. Follow these sequences as far back in time as possible. You may even arrive at the Big Bang! Give thanks. Now enjoy. It may take you 10 minutes to experience that little kiss of chocolate, but what happens as a result? Your anticipation has expanded and enhanced your desire.

While this short exercise is commonly used to introduce mindful awareness as an alternative to the habitual, mindless way of eating, it also applies as an alternative to the routine way of engaging in sex. The solution is to slow down, focus on that thing, and find joy in the moment. I know. To an OC, slowing down borders on sacrilege. And OCs believe that multiprocessing, multitasking, and productivity are virtues. Society has long espoused the message: *"Get as productive as possible in the least amount of time so that you can enjoy yourself."* Of course, there's always more to do and too little time to do it. The result is that there's never any joy to be had.

Here's the scientific truth: multiprocessing doesn't comport well with how the mind works. The mind can only focus on one thing at a time. Therefore, if you want to focus on two things, your mind gives 50 percent of your focused attention to one subject and 50 percent to the other. While multiprocessing is a myth, the effects of distraction have real-world consequences. For example, distractions from smartphones and emails drive down IQ.[34] Not very smart of our smartphones, eh?!?

As Sheri tells her story, she would be having sex when a notification chime on her phone causes her attention to shift away from the intimate moment, and she becomes overwhelmed with mind chatter: *"Who is that? Is it urgent? What if it's an emergency? What if it's about my mom or dad? Jeez, I wish we'd hurry up here so that I can check my phone."* There's only one job when you're having sex—to have a good time. Thinking about anything else will rob you of the pleasure potential.

The Raisin Exercise is a reminder that finding enjoyment in something like sex requires focused attention and freedom from distraction. If you're aware that you're prone to distraction and have a mind determined to multi-process or multitask, this exercise will be challenging, but that's good. Make it easier on yourself by intentionally removing distractions such as phones and pets, and turn off the TV. (Better yet, remove the TV from the bedroom!)

Use Your Mind as a Tool

The bulk of my work helping patients make nice with naughty is educating them on how their minds work. You'll find more enjoyment, pleasure, and fuel for your fire of desire by using your mind as a tool versus your mind using you as one. Whenever you feel stressed, that's evidence that your mind is using you as a tool. Conversely, there's no stress when you're no longer being worked by your mind-chatter. There's the reality check for you then: if there's stress, you're the tool!

---

[34] Rosen, Christine (Spring, 2008). *The Myth of Multi-Tasking.* The New Atlantis. Retrieved from https://www.thenewatlantis.com/publications/the-myth-of-multitasking

For example, many OCs struggle with a sense of unworthiness. Their egos tell them that they can resolve that feeling by striving for more, which leads to various forms of hoarding of safety and security. Your mind quickly becomes dissatisfied with what you have and focuses its sights on the next thing, dwelling in the future and not the now, believing that acquiring that thing will bring the contentment you think is necessary. The ego is quite seductive this way.

A sure-fire way for the ego to let go of you is to bring your attention to one or more of the five senses. If you're prone to distraction, focus on what you can see, touch, hear, smell, or taste. You may even find it helpful to draw from one of the most common grounding techniques for anxiety, the 5-4-3-2-1 Method.

When in an intimate moment with your partner, focus on and acknowledge:

- **Five** things you can see: your partner's silhouette, their eyes, the room, the candle flickering, etc.
- **Four** things you can physically feel: your partner's skin, their hair, the sheets, your skin, etc.
- **Three** things you can hear: the sounds of lovemaking, the fan, the flicker from the candlewick.
- **Two** things you can smell: the scent of the candle, the scent of your partner.
- **One** thing you can taste: the wine lingering in your mouth.

This exercise is the ultimate in being present, in being in the flow of the now moment; focusing on and loving what *is* rather than what *is not*; and finding joy, happiness, and satisfaction. It forces your ego to release you from believing that your joy can only be found in the next moment and that you're not deserving of it or it's not deserving of you right now.

If you find your mind wandering, you can reclaim your power by voicing your experience to your partner and being authentic in stating the obvious. *"My mind is distracted right now. You might have noticed. I want to focus on us and on my experience of being with you. I'm going to get a drink of water and come back. Don't move!"* This simple acknowledgment helps put any perceived distance or distraction into context. In addition, your awareness of the distraction is evidence of your being mindful where you're now observing your mind's distracted state. You've separated yourself from your ego. How cool is that!?!

Grasping and Wanting: Painful Desires

A significant structure of the mind is its tendency toward unhealthy forms of wanting, also known as grasping. Grasping, clinging, and attachment essentially mean psychologically holding on to some idea of *"This is mine"* or, *"This is me. This is who I am."* It's a state of mind characterized by never being content or satisfied with the present and wanting the moment to be different than what it is. Buddhist philosophers and practitioners have long realized that the ego's grasping for something different is at the core of human suffering.

As I described in Chapter 6, *healthy wanting* moves us toward our values. *Unhealthy wanting*, or grasping, is being desirous of the next moment more than that of the now. This phenomenon is powerful among OCs when that trait is entrenched in our moral certitude. The mind makes you believe that grasping is necessary to have the level of safety and security that you feel is needed to live a happy life when in reality, you're being prodded by your ego to attach to an erroneous and unhealthy ideal. Sexual perfectionism is a perfect example of grasping for or clinging to an ideal that can become detrimental to your sexual and intimate relationships.

Another dimension of grasping is rigid planning. OCs are great planners. Compulsive rehearsal, premeditation, and preparation are common traits among OC people. Now, there's nothing inherently wrong with planning, but what can happen is that an attachment can develop to a particular plan and outcome. It can be painful, though, when reality starts to move in a direction that doesn't align with the plan and its intended effect.

Take Patrick. He has mentally rehearsed what he wants to have happen when engaging in sex with his partner. He's created a sort of *destination addiction* whereby he fixates on the belief that happiness is in some destination or some other moment than this one. His partner's spontaneity and playfulness throw a wrench into Patrick's proceedings, and he shuts down, having grasped and clung so tightly to the desired outcome that he can't allow any other thoughts in or leave room to question his ego's grasp on him.

Loving Kindness Meditation

Loving Kindness Meditation is a broadly accepted self-care technique often used to reduce stress and anxiety and enhance well-being. Those who regularly practice it can increase their capacity for self-acceptance, forgiveness, more meaningful relationships with others, and more.

This meditation typically begins in a similar fashion as described in the Raisin Exercise above. Sit comfortably with good posture. Bring your awareness to your breathing: inhaling, exhaling; in breath, out breath. Notice the rise and fall of your breath with each interval. After a series of intervals, call forth an image of someone who truly has your best interest at heart. This person can be from your past or present: a mentor, a family member, a teacher, a friend, or a colleague. See their face in your mind's eye. Imagine them sitting before you, smiling, warmly looking back at you. Imagine them wishing you to be happy and fulfilled. With each inhale, take in the love they emanate. Allow your experience of warmth and positivity to grow as well.

Using the words of the Buddhist nun, teacher, and author, Pema Chödrön, repeat to yourself, *"May you be free of suffering and the root of suffering; may you enjoy happiness and the root of happiness."* Allow this experience to open the heart. Let that experience build and sit with it for a moment.

Send those loving feelings to yourself from that place and space of an open heart: *"May I be free of suffering and the root of suffering; may I enjoy happiness and the root of happiness."* Again, sit with that feeling. Observe it. Notice whether any psychological and/or emotional obstacles arise. Sit with it; observe it. Breathe loving-kindness in their direction.

After a few moments, you can move to imagine someone whom you know very little, perhaps your grocery store cashier, a co-worker in another department, or your neighbor from down the street. Repeat to yourself, *"May they be free of suffering and the root of suffering; may they enjoy happiness and the root of happiness."* Later, you can move toward sending loving-kindness to those who've harmed you. *"May they be free of suffering and the root of suffering; may they enjoy happiness and the root of happiness."*

With an open-hearted, non-reactive, non-judgmental presence, you can see into the nature of the anger or grief for whatever it is. And in the seeing, in the embracing of it, and knowing it, the anger, unhappiness, or anxiety attenuates, weakens, and dissolves, very much like touching a soap bubble or writing on water. This is your ego letting go of you.

The Loving Kindness Meditation is not easy for many who've felt and feared criticism most of their lives. It can also be challenging and sometimes leads to resistance for those unfamiliar with this level of giving and receiving love. Yet, even in the smallest of ways initially, practicing it could lead you to bloom a greater love and compassion for yourself.

Forgive me if I sound a bit woo-woo for a moment here, but you were born out of love. Not necessarily the love of your parents (hopefully so), but from the universe's love. Isn't it amazing that every atom that makes up your body began its cosmic journey at the moment of the big bang and has traveled throughout time and space to condense down into the form that we call You! Of all the possibilities, those atoms came together to form *you*. You *are* the miracle the universe manifested and are deserving of your loving kindness.

This atoms-coursing-through-the-universe stuff may seem like something otherworldly, but it illustrates the connectedness of it all and our rightful place to be in the now-moment and give and receive love. Loving kindness for yourself and for others is a product of mindfulness. The problem is that many people, OCs in particular, have difficulty slowing their minds down to a speed that can allow for self-reflection and recognizing and accepting ourselves for who we are and not the person our egos want us to be. Yet, you've picked up this book and you've hung in there with me thus far. It tells me that your ego is slowly letting go of you.

The Power of Mindfulness

If you've come this far, you're finished with being controlled by your fears and anxieties, and you're beginning to understand what it means to express and find sexual enjoyment. You now have the courage and resolve to know the truth of what you're thinking and feeling, to experience your wide-awake mind, and to have the open heart to follow what your unencumbered thoughts are telling you.

The psychologist Jack Kornfield offers one simple yet effective tool for putting a pin in the map of our true selves. He provides his methodology, RAIN (Recognition, Acceptance, Investigation, and Non-Identification), as a helpful tool for experiencing the transformational power of mindfulness in a general sense.[35] We'll apply Kornfield's model to our goal of making nice with naughty and use the four elements in his approach as an exercise to help you slow your mind down and become the observer and fair witness of the now moment.

---

[35] Kornfield, Jack (2022). *RAIN: Principles for Mindful Transformation*. Retrieved from https://jackkornfield.com/doing-the-buddhas-practice/.

So often, you'll hear OCs say, *"My mind races a million miles a minute. I just can't slow my mind down."* To experience the power of mindfulness, you need to pump the brakes and get control over the ego-driven rush of thoughts and feelings. Let's return to Sheri's and Patrick's stories at the onset of this chapter and apply Dr. Kornfield's RAIN methodology to help Sheri find a way to quell her intrusive thoughts and be fully in the moment with her partner and offer Patrick a means by which he can open his mind and discover the passion awaiting him by accepting his partner's invitation to be spontaneous and playful with her.

Recognize the Moment for What It Is

As an OC, you likely find moments when you feel stuck sexually and cannot get to where and what you want. An important, qualifying aspect of mindfulness is being non-resistant to the present moment. That begins with the recognition of the situation for what it is. Recognition starts the minute you focus your attention on whatever thoughts, emotions, feelings, or sensations arise right in the here and now.

Sheri's recognition is that she's multiprocessing at a most intimate time and that her mind-chatter is compelling her to think of all the things that she needs to do. Just her recognition—*"I'm not present right now. My mind has taken me somewhere else"*—is the necessary first step. As a fair witness of yourself, slow down for a moment and recognize your thoughts and feelings for what they are with understanding and compassion.

Patrick's recognition is that of his partner's desire for spontaneity and his rigid attachment to his rehearsed sequence for sex, which doesn't allow any room for spontaneity or playfulness. Patrick's recognition is that his inflexibility and emotional retreat when his partner gets playful is his ego arguing with the reality of the moment, which is never a winning proposition. As Byron Katie puts it, *"When you argue with reality, you'll lose, but only one hundred percent of the time."*

Accept the Reality of the Moment

By first recognizing the moment for what it is and that life is as it is, you've now opened yourself to accepting the reality of the moment and receiving it without harsh judgment of yourself. Non-acceptance would be Patrick arguing with reality by thinking, *"I'm not going to participate in this moment with her. It's not where I wanted to go,"* then shutting down because events didn't turn out as planned. As soon as Patrick accepts the *is-ness* of the moment—recognizing his partner's invitation to play—he says *yes* to her asking and becomes open to engaging in whatever it is that she wants to get into.

Acceptance allows you to relax and be open to the facts before you. It's a necessary next step and flows from recognition because, with recognition, there can come resistance, a wish that it weren't so or wasn't true. With recognition *and* acceptance, you're acknowledging and welcoming the truth of the moment for what it is.

Sheri's acceptance is her acknowledgment of and allowance for her mind that leans toward multitasking. She's not judging her thoughts, just recognizing and giving credence to how her mind works when she's trying to be sexually intimate with her partner while focusing on her unfinished projects, domestic chores, etc.

Sheri has accepted her propensity to engage in this kind of running to-do list, trying to tackle things she can't possibly deal with in a horizontal position. She's not judging her distractions. That makes matters worse by creating yet another mental obstacle diverting her attention away from the moment. It's either judge or ignore because once you begin to judge, you're allowing yourself to be drawn into that distraction, which empowers your ego to command your thoughts. Instead, Sheri simply recognizes and accepts that this is how her mind works.

Investigate with Thoughtfulness

There are times when merely working through the first two steps of recognizing and accepting is enough to quell your fears and anxieties and connect you with the present moment. At other times, your intention to recognize the moment for what it is and allow it to pass by not holding onto it is not enough. Simply pausing to ask, *"What is happening inside me, and how is my body reacting?"* might initiate recognition and acceptance of what is. Still, in this third step of the investigation, you engage in a more active and pointed examination of yourself, primarily your physical self.

Earlier, I introduced the 5-4-3-2-1 Method to bring you closer to what you're actually doing in your now moment. For example, when you're in the shower, are you really in the shower, or are you thinking about the phone call you need to make as soon as you've dried off? However, if you're really present in your shower, you're listening to the water running and feeling its temperature on your back. You're smelling the fragrance of your shampoo and soap. You're fully engaged in taking your shower. Many people tend not to peer deeply enough into their experiences and miss the pleasure of not only their showers but so many other happenings in their lives.

Sheri may recognize and accept that she's multitasking while engaging in sex with her partner. Still, unless the physical feeling of her multitasking and sexual experience are brought into her consciousness, her beliefs and emotions will continue to control and overwhelm her experience when she's with her partner and deprive her of being in the moment with him.

In this step, Sheri might ask herself, *"What most wants my attention?"* Or, *"What does this feeling want from me, and how am I experiencing this in my body?"* Sheri also wants to bring front and center into her consciousness the physical sensation of having sex with her partner. She does this by focusing on the reality of what it feels like have his weight on her body, his breathing, and the fullness of his penis inside of her. These are the different ways Sheri can bring attention back to the now-moment.

Patrick's investigation of his partner's desire to be playful and his reaction to it would be along the lines of what he would be doing if he were living out the moment according to his values. He wouldn't want to be seen as someone who's not playful. His inquiry would put him in touch with his body, and his becoming rigid when his partner approaches him spontaneously and touches him. His noticing the physical sensation of every muscle in his body becoming stiff except for the muscles of his penis can allow him then to investigate the feeling of letting some of those muscles relax and become a bit more playful with Sheri, regardless of how awkward it may feel. To this last point, many people, with OCs in particular, may think that being a good lover means having confidence, which means never feeling awkward. In reality, the willingness to have awkwardness be present and still move toward what you want is the truer display of confidence. Why argue with reality?

Don't Identify the Moment as *You*

Remember my raising "self-as-context" as a positive viewpoint from which we observe our thoughts and feelings and the psychological space in which they can move within our consciousness? Non-identification reinforces (a) the concept of you being your sky, the sentinel of your world, and (b) that the thoughts and feelings you're experiencing are the passing fronts that form your mind-chatter.

Your recognition, acceptance, and investigation have led you to the freedom of non-identification. Your sense of who you are is not attached to or defined by any restricting thoughts or feelings that only tend to create dependence, anxiety, inauthenticity, and more. Buddhism calls non-identification "The abode of the awakening, the end of clinging, true peace, nirvana." You can experience sexual enjoyment and fulfillment because your fears and illusions no longer bind you.

In practicing non-identification, we question every experience by asking, *"Is this who I really am?"* Sheri's non-identification is in her recognizing that she's multitasking when she's intimate with her partner and accepting, without judgment or awfulizing, that her mind leans in that direction. She brings her consciousness back to the now-moment. Sheri's no longer identifying with multitasking as "me."

Patrick's non-identification is in recognizing that his partner's spontaneity and playfulness conflict with his rigid attachment to his sequence for sex and causes him to freeze. His acceptance is being open to his partner's invitation to play and being willing to investigate the sensation of letting go and pushing through any awkwardness—the definition of a confident sex partner. With this reasoning, Patrick's ego dissipates and releases him. He no longer identifies as someone who's not willing to be open-minded and flexible.

Slow your thoughts down long enough to recognize the moment for what it is. Accept its reality without judgment of yourself or others. Be the sentinel of your being, engage in a more active and critical examination of your fears and anxieties, and free yourself from letting your mind-chatter define you. Just as we've explored and practiced in this chapter, your mindfulness can tame the monkey and allow you to be in the moment, open, and wanting with your heart to make nice with naughty.

EXERCISE: CRAFTING YOUR FLEXIBLE FANTASY

For too long, your rules-based mind-chatter has kept you from engaging and making nice with naughty, and your ego has repeated your anxiety mantra or mantras for too long: *"I have to feel X, first, before I can enjoy sex."* Here are just some examples of rules that OCs believe must be met first to have an anxious-free mind:

"The kitchen has to be clean before I can have sex."
"Sex can only happen on weekends."
"I first have to feel trust and confidence in my partner."
"I have to have an erection first."
"It's not sex if I don't orgasm."

What has *your* mind-chatter tried to convince you that must first exist in your thoughts, in your partner's behavior, or in your environment before you can experience sexual enjoyment and fulfillment?

1.
2.
3.
4.
5.

Notice how easy it is for your mind to create rules? You see, your mind, like my mind, thrives on certainty. In this case, your head says, *"Hey, me! If I have these certainties first, then I'll surely not experience negative feelings in the future."* Unfortunately, there is no certainty. There never was or will be a certainty. The most you'll ever have is pseudo-certainty—the false sense that you know how the future will play out.

However, you can choose to behave differently and act in a way consistent with your vision of a future you want for yourself. In other words, you can be mentally adaptable, thus visualizing, choosing, and practicing those preferred behaviors even when those old feelings of insecurity, fear, and uncertainty persist within you. Try it.

What Is Your Flexible Fantasy?

If you were to fantasize about your sex life, what would you want that life to be? Use the space below (use extra paper if needed!) to craft a sexual fantasy that reflects what's important to you, absent of all the anxiety and fear that has ever informed your fantasies of sex and sexuality in the past. Imagine being in your most enjoyable, most comfortable place for sex with your partner. What would that experience be like? Keep in mind that there is no right or wrong way to do this. Whatever you experience is your experience.

| |
| |

Now, imagine that you're engaging in sex and begin experiencing that mind-chatter that you typically experience from the list above. Now imagine changing those feelings of anxiety to simple disappointment and frustration. How would you dispute each of the anxiety mantras you've listed above? What new experience would emerge for you and your partner as a result?

1.
2.

3.
4.
5.

CHAPTER 9
VICTIM TO VICTORIOUS

"Forgiveness is giving up all hope for a better past."

— Lily Tomlin

"It's hard for me to enjoy sex. It makes me anxious. I'm distracted by thoughts and images of my past. I wish I could just get over it, but it feels like I need to heal from my trauma before I can enjoy it. Frankly, and I hate to admit it, I'm not even sure I'm all that motivated to do the work. I mean, my relationship with sex now is more of a 'take sex or leave it.' I also know, though, that it's a wedge between my partner and me. I recognize it's unfair to him; he didn't hurt me, but my feelings need to be recognized."

Tens of millions share Sara's anxious feelings about sex. She is one of a community of people who have experienced sexual trauma. The National Sexual Violence Resource Center reports that more than 80 percent of women in the United States have faced sexual harassment or assault at some point in their lives; one-in-five have experienced completed or attempted rape. Most sexual violence occurs at the hands of a family member, intimate partner, or acquaintance. While most perpetrators are male, eight to 17 percent of sexual offenders are female and could be one's mother, aunt, cousin, or babysitter.[36]

---

[36] Haines, Staci (May 28, 1999). *The Survivor's Guide to Sex: How to Have an Empowered Sex Life After Child Sexual Abuse.* Cleis Press. Retrieved from https://www.amazon.com/Survivors-Guide-Sex-Empowered-Sexual/dp/1573440795/ref=sr_1_1?crid=ZUI9K3FGPN1R&keywords=the+survivors+guide+to+sex&qid=1656503618&sprefix=the+survivor+s+guide+to+sex%2Caps%2C202&sr=8-1.

Another source for statistics, The Rape, Abuse, and Incest National Network (RAINN), indicates that 93 percent of sexual offenders are known to the victim. Of them, 59 percent are acquaintances, and 34 percent are family members. Only seven percent are strangers.[37] Read that again: only seven percent are strangers.

For many, male or female, the familiar nature of one's abuser is particularly traumatizing. Abuse within these intimate relationships can shake the core of one's sense of safety and security and interfere with an ability to develop trust. A significant dilemma facing those who've experienced sexual trauma is, as Staci Haines writes in *The Survivor's Guide to Sex: How to Have an Empowered Sex Life After Child Sexual Abuse*, "the need to survive *and* the need to be connected and loved."[38] Typically, these needs of survival and connectedness operate in harmony, but for those who've been sexually traumatized, particularly children, these needs can compete with one another.

Let me explain. Whenever you face danger, the reptilian and mammalian parts of your brain activate, and it all comes down to one question: *"How do I survive this?"* Sexual abuse at the hands of someone familiar complicates matters. You have this experience that feels dangerous and wrong, yet the perpetrator is someone with whom you may also feel deeply attached. Moreover, some survivors report their bodies responding to the sexual stimulation with either genital engorgement or an orgasm. (These responses simply reflect the body doing what it was designed to do in the face of particular stimulation and doesn't necessarily reflect one's subjective experience of consent

---

[37] RAINN (Rape, Abuse & Incest National Network). *Children and Teens: Statistics*. Retrieved from https://www.rainn.org/statistics/children-and-teens.

[38] Haines, ibid.

or pleasure.) The complexity of factors can become even more confusing when one's abuser holds a caregiver position over the survivor (e.g., parent/step-parent, grandparent, uncle, teacher, minister, babysitter, etc.).

I am an adult survivor of childhood sex abuse. The abuse didn't just happen once or a few times at the hands of one person, but rather multiple times involving multiple people, including family members. For readers who've experienced sexual abuse, I share that lived experience with you, and I empathize with you. I understand first-hand the confusion around sex and sexuality that comes about from sexual abuse. Without question, the abuse impacted me, as I'm sure yours impacted you as well. My experience of abuse, however, never defined me. I seemed to have intuitively known that *I* defined the experience. This psychological realization is what allows me, and can enable you, to transition from victim to victorious. This transition is essential for anyone who's experienced sexual abuse, feels limited by that abuse, and yet yearns to make nice with naughty.

A major component of the transition from victim to victorious is an openness to examine and question your thoughts about your experience. To that end, some may wonder whether the suggestions I'm putting forth in this chapter constitute *gaslighting*. Gaslighting[39] is a form of psychological manipulation in which the abuser attempts to sow seeds of self-doubt and confusion in the victim's mind around the validity of their own experience. Gaslighters seek to gain power and control over others by distorting reality and forcing victims to question their judgment and intuition and convince them that the gaslighter's view of reality is truer.

---

[39] The popular notion of gaslighting comes from the 1944 moving, *Gaslight* starring Charles Boyer and Ingrid Bergman in which Boyer's character marries Bergman's character. Boyer tries to convince Bergman that she's losing her mind by, among other things, arranging for the gaslights in their 19th century house to dim without being touched.

I'm mentioning this because I want to be transparent about my intent. My book discusses the approaches you can use to overcome psychological obstacles interfering with interpersonal connectedness and sexual enjoyment. To that end, I aim to help you reduce your suffering, identify *your* truth that's free of cognitive biases and distortions, and allow *you* to choose behaviors that are consistent with *your* values. Whereas gaslighting is about diminishing personal agency, the methods I refer to in this chapter (e.g., REBT, RO DBT, and self-inquiry as espoused by Byron Katie) are about maximizing personal agency.

When working with survivors of sexual abuse who experience echoes of history within their current sexual and intimate relationships, I aim to help them move from victim to victorious by focusing on what they do have control over: their thoughts and behaviors. Abusers' manipulation impacts how you come to see yourself and shapes the nature of your mind-chatter. The first betrayal occurs when the abuser attacks your personhood; the final betrayal is when you believe them.

The impact of sexual abuse, however, can wax and wane. Some find sex relatively easy and enjoyable early on in a relationship. You may have found yourself quite receptive and excited about sex during the early phase of the courtship. However, many of my patients report that this excitement doesn't last very long. They eventually come to me with questions about why their desire for sex diminished. They develop sexual perfectionism as the emotional bonds intensify within their relationship. Some report flashbacks that remind them of their loving, familial bond with the family member who abused them. Naturally, these mental hurdles block one's pursuit of the sexual freedom that they're looking for.

The Path from Victim to Victorious

I believe that the story we tell ourselves about our trauma is the biggest impediment to finding enjoyment and fulfillment in our sexual life and intimate relationships. My intent with this chapter is to move you from that victim narrative to a victorious healing narrative. What I seek to do is to increase your personal agency through your self-inquiry and self-acceptance. To that end, this chapter has two parts: the first is intended to help you unearth unhealthy negative feelings, expose the myth of self-esteem, and show how the ego thrives on the victimhood personality.

Part two turns the page from understanding the victim to becoming the victorious with your own healing narrative through accepting yourself and forgiving past hurts in order to heal, by engaging in the five exercises that support post-traumatic growth, and finally by your narrating how you will live out your goal for making nice with naughty. At the end of the chapter, I encourage you to participate in a mindfulness practice called the Forgiveness Exercise to stimulate self-inquiry and find new language that will enable you to move beyond the trauma narrative that shackles you to that history.

I recognize that not everyone reading this book has experienced sexual trauma in their life, yet you share the same goal of making nice with naughty once again in your life, or for the first time. While this chapter may not speak directly to you, you may still know someone—a family member or close friend—who has experienced sexual abuse in their lifetime. To that end, the material and exercises shared in this chapter can be valuable for you for it will add a new dimension to your understanding of their experiences.

With that path and intent in mind, let's now delve further into Sara's story. After processing with Sara her experience with flashbacks and her anxieties when having sex with her partner, I offered, *"My focus, Sara, is to ultimately help you continue on your path from victim to victorious that frees you from the effects of your past."*

"What do you mean 'continue'?" she asked.

"Well, let's look at reality, and you know how much I love reality." We chuckle together. *"If you're here, in this moment, you've survived everything that's ever happened to you, right? I mean, you've not died from any decision that you've made, correct?"*

Sara laughed, *"Yeah, I'm here."*

I went on, *"All the decisions you've made and actions you've taken have been the right ones. How do I know? Again, because you're here, in this moment with me. You've made it here—the only moment that exists. That sounds like the path to victory to me."*

Sara reflects for a moment and responds, *"My mind says, 'If I had only made different choices, then I'd be happier, healthier, and more fulfilled.'"*

"Those are some seductive thoughts, aren't they?" I asked. *"They make you think that there is some Sara in some alternative universe who's living her best life because she seemed to have avoided the abuse altogether or made different choices along the way that reduced the impact of the abuse.*

"However, those thoughts are just forms of mental-masturbation. Let's look at reality again. Even if there was this Sara in this alternative universe living her best life, what relevance does that have for you living your life today? In fact, the more disparate your life is from that imagined Sara, and the more you compare your life to hers, the more you suffer.

"Again, don't take my word for it. Just look at your own experience. But, if we come back to this moment, this life, with you right here, right now, sitting in my office, what do you notice?"

"It is true; I have been doing better," she reflected. *"Although I still have thoughts about my uncle, I'm in a real relationship for the first time, maybe in my lifetime. I'm just not motivated or enthused about having sex now. I did initially when my partner and I first met, but we're closer now, and these anxieties are surfacing from my past and holding me back. I feel for my partner because I know he has desires."*

Sara feels stuck, and the trauma narrative plaguing her thoughts is the obstacle. That is why she is not enjoying sex with her partner and questions whether she can change the narrative. However, what she's discovering is that her hurt feelings and distressing thoughts about the events are what's disturbing and disrupting her life now and not the event itself. Let's explore that further.

Unhealthy Negative Feelings

In Chapter 5, I introduced the innovative and practical approach of Dr. Albert Ellis. I outlined the core components of his Rational Emotive Behavior Therapy (REBT), which he termed the ABCs of emotional disturbance: the **A**ctivating Event, when a perceived threat happens in the environment around you; your core **B**eliefs, which describe your thoughts attached to the activating event; and the **C**onsequences, which are your emotional and behavioral reactions to your thoughts about the situation that activates the event for you. The basic concept underlying the ABCs is that external circumstances do not cause disturbances (e.g., anxiety, anger, etc.) but that irrational beliefs do; and that we have the power to change those beliefs in order to have a different affective response.

Humans are full of cognitive biases and errors. One of the prominent ones observed in psychotherapy among distressed persons is, *"I'm [insert feeling word, such as anxious or depressed] because of [insert event]."* However, as the Stoics found two millennia ago, it's not the events that disturb us; it's our beliefs, attitudes, and philosophy about the events that distract, disrupt, and intrude on us.

Traumatic experiences are atrocious, sad, and regrettable, and often *very* harmful. Of course, it's appropriate to feel strongly about the offense. However, your thought choices determine whether you'll experience healthy negative feelings or unhealthy and maladaptive negative feelings. Sadness about your traumatic incident is a healthy negative feeling; despair about the experience is not. Unhealthy or maladaptive negative emotions obstruct your progress toward goals that are meaningful to you. Feelings of hopelessness, worry, or despondency, as example, are inconsistent with developing greater physical intimacy with your partner. In short, maladaptive negative emotions rarely lead to a greater connection between you and your partner.

When people develop unhealthy negative feelings, they're prone to harboring maladaptive beliefs, such as *"I'll never heal from this," "All sex is bad,"* or *"Men just want one thing."* Many of these unhealthy feelings may include self-blame that stems from irrational beliefs such as you being the cause of the assault or that you should have acted differently when the abuse happened.

That negative or irrational deductive reasoning often leads to a string of unfounded beliefs, each dependent upon the first maladaptive belief, including, *"Who would ever really want me?"* or *"If someone wants me, they only want me sexually. They're not really interested in me,"* and *"I'm undeserving of real love."*

REBT endeavors to cut that string, freeing you to accept yourself without any conditions. This therapeutic approach brings you to the realization that you are separate from your anxieties, that you have strengths and weaknesses, that you've made mistakes, and that you have flaws. **Yet none of this defines you.** Through unconditional self-acceptance, you accept that you've been hurt, yet acknowledge that the event doesn't portray who you are. Traumatic events may have happened to you, but your personhood is not damaged.

The Flaws about Self-Esteem

I would like to contrast unconditional self-acceptance with the concept of *self-esteem*—the darling of so many therapists and self-help gurus. I believe self-esteem is flawed because it is inherently self-evaluative and conditional. It implies, *"When I'm doing good, I can feel good about myself; but if I'm doing badly, I risk feeling bad about myself."* Self-esteem forces you to seek evidence of your own worth. That means, when most people talk about self-esteem, they're really talking about *borrowed-esteem*—the dopamine boost you get from internalizing others' positive perceptions of you. One of the flaws is, when the well runs dry, those seeking self-esteem may question their worth again.

Overcontrolled people whose tendency is to be highly engaged in social comparison are particularly susceptible to borrowed-esteem. I'm not saying self-esteem is inherently wrong; after all, it's our nature to want to be a part of a tribe. It's a preferred human experience to be accepted by others. However, we question our relevance when we demand it as a function of our sense of being and don't receive it.

The reality is—and hold onto yourself because I'm about to hand you some Dr. Murray realness—you have no worth. Hear me out now. Don't close the book yet. What I mean is that things, you included, do not have inherent value. Instead, humans project value onto things. For example, if you own a home, you might think, *"My house is worth $X."* Of course, your house isn't worth X. Your house's value depends on what another person is willing to pay for it. You might argue and think that your home is worth more than what someone is willing to pay, but unless you have a buyer for that price, it's not worth what you think. In short, the thing's value isn't *IN* the thing; humans project value onto it.

In a similar sense, self-esteem is a measure of one's worth. And when you buy into the myth of self-esteem, you're constantly looking for evidence of your self-worth, or if you're prone to a victimhood personality (a topic I will cover shortly), you might be looking for evidence of your lack of worth with maladaptive thoughts such as, *"I'm undeserving of this."*

Consequently, the myth of self-esteem perpetuates a lot of unhappiness and is a significant source of suffering for many. For example, many people are told, *"You should love yourself."* That sounds all warm and fuzzy, doesn't it? Yet let's do a thought experiment. How does it feel inside to believe the thought, *"I should love myself"* when, in fact, you don't love yourself? If you're like most people, you feel worse inside. Love is immutable; it's not subject to others' perceptions. Another way of understanding the nature of love is through acceptance. When you accept somebody just as they are, including yourself, that's real love. Why is that important to this idea of victim to victorious? Because nothing in the universe, including others' perceptions of you, can diminish who you are.

Now, this will sound woo-woo, and it's only the second time in this book that I've gone to the woo-woo. The other was in Chapter 3 when I shared that *you* are not your mind-chatter; you are that which observes the mind-chatter. In this instance, the unconventional belief that I hold is that the energy that sustains your body (i.e., lifeforce) is who you *really* are beyond the ego. This energy has existed since the beginning of time. How do we know? Because energy cannot be created or destroyed (i.e., the first law of thermodynamics). Therefore, if the energy that sustains your body has always existed and *will* always exist, then there's nothing in the universe that can diminish the *you* that you are behind your ego.

Byron Katie calls this energy *love*. She writes,

"Love is what you are already. Love doesn't seek anything. It's already complete. It doesn't want, doesn't need, has no shoulds. It already has everything it wants. It already is everything it wants, just the way it wants it. So, when I hear people say that they love someone and want to be loved in return, I know they're not talking about love. They're talking about something else."[40]

What is this something else? It's the ego/personality. Yet, the ego is temporary as well and will dissolve the moment you take your last

---

[40] Katie, Byron & Katz, Michael (November 28, 2006). *I Need Your Love – Is That True?: How to Stop Seeking Love, Approval, and Appreciation and Start Finding Them Instead*, p 7. Harmony Publishing. Retrieved from https://www.amazon.com/Need-Your-Love-Approval-Appreciation/dp/0307345300/ref=asc_df_0307345300/?tag=hyprod-20&linkCode=df0&hvadid=312674808447&hvpos=&hvnetw=g&hvrand=8654632277138145350&hvpone=&hvptwo=&hvqmt=&hvdev=c&hvdvcmdl=&hvlocint=&hvlocphy=9010811&hvtargid=pla-489337318527&psc=1.

breath on this blue marble; the energy will transform into something else. Religion provides frameworks and belief systems for understanding what that something else is; science simply tells us that the energy transforms. Taken in its totality, the bottom line is that no abuse has ever happened to you or misfortunes have ever come to you that diminished your being, no matter how powerfully painful that abuse.

Katie offers another invaluable nugget:

"Seeking love keeps you from the awareness that you already have it—that you are it."[41]

Unconditional self-acceptance occurs when there is no rating of the self. It acknowledges that being human means being fallible, erring, and misbehaving. While self-esteem requires you to rate your personhood, unconditional self-acceptance requires you to rate your behavior against your goals and whether your actions are moving you toward what you want.

Let's apply Ellis' ABC model of emotional disturbance that I introduced earlier in the chapter to Sara's situation. You may even parallel and reflect on your traumatic experience as I walk through this process with Sara. I start with confirming why she's here as an initial step on her pathway from victim to victorious. I ask, *"What's your goal, Sara? What do you want to be different in your sexual and intimate relationship with your partner?"*

---

[41] Katie, Byron & Mitchell, Stephen (December 7, 2021). *Loving What Is. Revised Edition: Four Questions That Can Change Your Life*, p 243. Harmony Publishing. Retrieved from https://www.amazon.com/Loving-What-Revised-Questions-Change/dp/0593234510/ref=asc_df_0593234510/?tag=hyprod-20&linkCode=df0&hvadid=509494905560&hvpos=&hvnetw=g&hvrand=138039235 48720416439&hvpone=&hvptwo=&hvqmt=&hvdev=c&hvdvcmdl=&hvlocint=&hvl ocphy=9010811&hvtargid=pla-1277450139760&psc=1&asin=0593234510&revisionId=&format=4&depth=1

The North Star I spoke of in Chapter 6 that reflects what's important to us and guides us in our attempts to live authentic lives is what I want Sara to keep foremost in her mind. In the context of this book, your goal is to make nice with naughty. In so many words, that's Sara's goal as well.

She speaks to it this way, *"Well, I want to be more intimate with my partner. More comfortable with him when we're having sex."*

"Okay, great," I reply and follow up with, *"And what do you think gets in the way of being able to do that? What event or situation activates the thoughts that trigger you?"*

Sara hesitates at first, then begins speaking to those things that set off her negative feelings, *"When my partner comes on to me for sex."*

I ask, *"And, what are your thoughts and beliefs when your partner approaches you for sex?"*

"I feel anxious and have intrusive thoughts about my uncle and what my uncle did to me." Sara goes on, *"Joe should want to wait to have sex with me until I'm no longer anxious or likely to have these memories. He should want to wait until I feel at ease. I need him to recognize that I have this trauma history. He has to remember that I was abused, and he has to respect my feelings."*

I ask Sara this next question to help make the connection for her, *"There's a lot there, Sara. What happens as a consequence of your beliefs?"*

"I'm distracted by my thoughts and feelings from the past. I also experience my partner as if he's on the other team. I ultimately push him away. Sometimes, though, I'm just ambivalent and let him finish. I check out. I can't enjoy myself when flooded with all these thoughts. I just wish I could enjoy my sex life like everyone else!"

You can see how distressing Sara's thoughts are to her. Let's take a closer look and see what might be happening here. Sara's ego is grappling with feeling relevant. Her ego is invested in the trauma narrative. Recall, however, that the ego isn't the enemy. The ego endeavors to protect her from painful memories and the possibility of abuse happening again. Nevertheless, the ego also causes Sara to behave and respond to her partner as if he's responsible. Her ego convinces her to blame him for causing her anxieties by not being more sensitive and more attentive to her having been hurt. The following section explores how we might better understand this phenomenon.

The Ego's Investment in Victimhood

Victimhood personality is characterized by a maladaptive need for recognition, difficulty empathizing with others, feelings of moral superiority, and a desire for vengeance. However, it's important to note that a victimhood personality can develop regardless of whether one experienced trauma or victimization. In either event, victimhood is a defense mechanism used to manage difficult life situations.

Consequently, the victimhood personality leads to a negative view of life and what's possible. The victimhood temperament drives people to avoid risk by viewing themselves as "weak, traumatized, and aggrieved." Moreover, those with a victimhood temperament feel threatened when anyone challenges their victimhood status. They often want to punish those who threaten their self-perception as a victim.[42] OCs, in particular, may be prone to lingering effects of trauma due to their heightened sensitivity to threat, hypervigilance, detailed focused processing (where the bigger picture is missed), perseveration, and general negative appraisal of life events.

We each experience life differently through the lenses we've acquired throughout our lives, regardless of temperament. How can we know this? Consider this: if a hundred people watch the same event, no one will have identical stories about that one shared experience.

---

[42] Gabay, Rahav & Hameiri, Boaz & Rubel-Lifschitz, Tammy & Nadler, Arie (2020). *The Tendency for Interpersonal Victimhood: The Personality Construct and its Consequences.* Personality and Individual Differences, Volume 165. Retrieved from https://doi.org/10.1016/j.paid.2020.110134.

There will always be something different in each person's recollection and beliefs about what happened. Likewise, our traumatic experiences and how they reverberate in our lives are primarily due to our beliefs about those experiences. As I'll share time and again in this chapter, as I do with my patients: the primary cause of anyone's unhappiness is rarely the situation but the thoughts about the situation.

In the context of OC temperament, OCs might even minimize their experience with statements such as *"I shouldn't have these troubles."* Yet once you are in a state of resistance to reality, you are experiencing suffering. Try this thought exercise here: how does it feel to believe the thought that you shouldn't have these troubles, yet you do? It feels heavy, doesn't it? The truth is, you do have these troubles. The question is, what are you going to do about it?

The ego is always looking for relevance, which we discovered with Sara. That means it tries to seduce you to focus on its agenda, which is typically past- or future-oriented, not on the now moment. It's unsurprising, then, that any interaction closely mirroring the abuse will be associated with the traumatic experience of the past or discomfort that might happen in the future. Even when one's sexual partner is loving and supportive, sex can become complicated for survivors because of their distressing thoughts of abuse.

Some men and women, for example, report confusion about their sexual identity due to their history of abuse. Others, overwhelmed or distracted by past thoughts, may experience dissociation or a lack of sensation, despite what would appear to be adequate stimulation. Some have even described their experience of sex as a numbness; others report physical and psychological rigidity when their partner approaches them sexually. Still others struggle with expressing preferences or desires to their partners, having experienced perpetrators who had no regard for body autonomy.

According to Dr. Lynch in RO DBT, the "Don't hurt me" responses are behaviors intended to block unwanted feedback or block requests to join in a community activity.[43] In the context of sexual and intimate relationships and for one who has experienced sexual abuse, these responses block unwanted sexual acts that remind the abused person of the incident. Some of the most common statements I hear are, *"My partner should respect my abuse history. Their expectations are hurting me. It's unfair that my history isn't taken into account. If they were a caring person, they would stop pressuring me to change."*

Not to make light of trauma in any sense, but "Don't hurt me" responses can be a form of social signaling to accentuate their suffering and sacrifice. Their responses demonstrate and remind others that the burden of abuse they carry is heavier than that of others. Some OCs may believe that their suffering is their "cross to bear" and that it's somehow just (which is also an illusion).

Some go to therapy so they don't have to change. They'll explain to others, *"Well, at least I'm going to therapy."* The learning here is, therapy doesn't make things happen, however; *you* do. Therapy is really what happens between sessions. Therapy occurs when you take lessons from your sessions and make changes to how you think and behave.

Maintaining the thoughts and behaviors consistent with the role of the victim keeps the trauma narrative alive. People either progress toward changing their sexual narrative, or they continue to do things that keep those narrative embers burning, such as, *"My partner should respect my abuse."* While it's true that people deserve respect, sometimes the demand to be respected inadvertently keeps them stuck in their victim story. Their rationalizing will often be similar to Sara's, *"I have to feel comfortable first before I can have sex."*

We can't force ourselves to stop feeling something just because the feeling is unpleasant, nor do humans have control over emerging

---

[43] Lynch (n 1), p 37.

thoughts. Consequently, your option is to focus on what you do have control over: your behavior and your relationship with your thoughts. In short, you have the power to change the trauma narrative and unchain yourself from your past, which is where our path with take us in part two of this chapter.

MOVING TOWARD THE HEALING NARRATIVE

"Do you want to have a pain-free life or a meaningful life?" That's a question I often ask my patients. Rarely have I ever heard any of them say, *"I'd rather have a pain-free life."*

People want a life of meaning and inherently see the value of trials and tribulations as a source of that meaning. As the adage goes, "You have to have a test to have a testimony." If your life were a constant state of comfort, you would realize that your life was dull and lacked any real meaning.

When you reflect and think of all the challenges you've faced in your life, the memories that stand out are those recalling the crucibles you overcame. What also stands out is how, each time, you dusted yourself off and progressed forward, guided by your values and goals. This underscores how important pain can be in helping us craft lives worth living.

A story that comes to mind is that of Leona who came to see me in emotional distress caused by intense negative self-talk of regret and embarrassment. She shared a recent experience where she mustered the courage to approach a colleague she liked, Brian, at a work party. She had never pursued a man before, having believed that only men were the ones who initiated dates, or the only ones who were supposed to. Nevertheless, Leona asked, and Brian accepted. They went out on a couple of low-key dates, and a few days following their most recent outing, which she found pleasant enough, he didn't feel a spark and wasn't interested in continuing to pursue her romantically.

During our session, Leona described how devastated and regretful she felt after taking the risk with him and being rejected. After validating her feelings, I asked, *"Do you want to have a pain-free life or a meaningful life? Because if you focus on the rejection, you're missing the real triumph here: your courageous act of breaking the rules, making nice with naughty, and pursuing someone you liked. That's victorious in my book!"*

Leona had been working with me on reducing the volume on her OC tendencies. She eventually recognized that her rule-following, orderly expectations limited her emotionally, psychologically, and romantically. She used the skills that she was developing and took a risk—a big risk, at that! While it's natural to want the huge risk to come with a huge reward (i.e., a long-term relationship with Brian), the *real* reward is that Leona learned something new about herself. She learned she can take risks and tolerate painful feelings when life doesn't unfold according to plan. She feels sad for being rejected, but she's not resisting reality and wallowing in despair.

Accept the Pain and Forgive

In contemplative psychology, there's an axiom:

PAIN x RESISTANCE = SUFFERING

Pain is the feeling of unpleasant physical sensation or emotion. *Resistance* is how the ego expresses itself through thoughts, beliefs, or behaviors to interfere with your accepting the reality of pain. Resistance can arise through various forms of struggle associated with that pain, such as denial, complaining, or victimhood. When pain is multiplied by resistance, the product is *suffering*.

It's also been said that suffering is the story you tell yourself about the pain you're experiencing. Buddhist philosophers illustrate this sentiment with two arrows to explain how resistance to reality brings greater suffering. The first arrow is the traumatic event that stabbed you, and the second arrow is the one you repeatedly stab yourself with by the resistance surrounding the trauma.

Leona and Sara experienced varying forms of pain. Leona experienced the rejection of a man with whom she took a massive risk in pursuing romantically; Sara experienced sexual assault by her uncle. These events, respectively, were their first arrows. The negative self-talk that ensued became their second arrows.

According to Ellis, "People traumatize themselves by the attitudes that they take toward traumatic events."[44] It's one thing to experience the pain of trauma; it's another how one constructs a story that frames the experience. If the story is full of *"shoulds"* and *"should nots"* or *"musts"* and *"must nots,"* there is an inherent argument with reality. Moreover, it can create a sense that the abused *"must change"* these bad things in their lives, which then brings about anxiety when things don't change according to their preferences.

Additionally, suffering can be sustained when there's a tendency toward a pessimistic, victimhood mindset. Ironically, those in a state of suffering can't help themselves. You see, people's behavior reflects the thoughts that preceded that behavior. Everything you do, you do because you believe a thought. If you've acquired a victimhood mindset, you believe every thought is consistent with that outlook; sometimes, those thoughts are incessant. You learn to take your thoughts less seriously by developing a mindfulness practice.

Overcontrolled people and those with a victimhood mindset often ruminate on past trauma—an endless loop of mind-chatter that they *should* have told someone, or *should* have received therapy, or *should* have taken a different approach, or *should have* listened to that advice, as examples. People get trapped in their victim story, which locks them in their past or compels them to dread their future. However, you're reading this book because you want to get off this endless loop and reclaim your life. Throughout this book, I've provided strategies for accepting your past. I review them here.

---

[44] Volpe, Joseph S. Ph.D. (2020). Trauma Response Profile: An Afternoon with Dr. Albert Ellis, Esteemed Member of the Academy's Board of Scientific and Professional Advisors. American Academy of Experts in Traumatic Stress. Retrieved from https://www.aaets.org/traumatic-stress-library/trauma-response-profile-an-afternoon-with-dr-albert-ellis-esteemed-member-of-the-academys-board-of-scientific-and-professional-advisors.

First, let me remind you that you're a survivor. You come from a long line of survivors. Every generation before you, spanning literally millions of years, survived long enough to procreate. Isn't that phenomenal?!? More, since you were born, you've survived everything that's ever happened to you. Therefore, you're truly a success story.

Every decision you've made along the way must have been right because you're alive in this moment, reading this book. Sure, your mind wants to say, *"But I'd prefer to have had a different experience living a different life where my trauma didn't happen."* Agreed. I'd prefer that too, for you and me. Yet we had that unfortunate experience and survived. The proof is in the pudding, as they say.

Secondly, acceptance happens at the moment you step out of the incessant stream of thought so that you can observe the mind-chatter rather than be a participant in the chatter. This is why developing a mindfulness practice has become so important to me and the patients I treat and may become important to you.

Yes, I still suffer. Yes, I still get caught up in my own mind-chatter. But with mindfulness, I spend less time suffering today than I did a year ago, five years ago, or ten years ago. Most of us will never entirely rid ourselves of suffering. Still, mindfulness is one tool to reduce its intensity so that you can navigate life with the least amount of suffering necessary. Mindfulness alone hasn't been enough for me, however. My patients and I have benefited from integrating another powerful approach—*The Work* of Byron Katie.

In Chapter 3, I introduced *The Work* by Katie and her powerful yet straightforward method of questioning mind-chatter, creating more space between you and your experiences, and opening your mind to potentially life-transforming insights.[45] *The Work* is the third method of cultivating acceptance. Consider revisiting Katie's approach to questioning specific thoughts that your ego has imposed on you,

---

[45] Katie (n 6), pp 17–21.

inspecting those thoughts to determine their truth, and turning your thoughts around to see if the opposite is true or truer than your assumptions.

Katie's approach helps you differentiate between truth and illusion of egoic mind-chatter. Recall that the truth always feels light—without exception—not heavy and stressful. As one patient said, *"If it's not light, it mustn't be right."* The truth is light because it reflects reality—a reality free from the mind's judgments. When I talk about acceptance, I'm talking about accepting truth—accepting reality. *The Work* helps you to discern between truth and illusion. "I'm responsible for the abuse." If you go inside and ask whether that thought feels light or heavy, you'll immediately recognize its weightiness. The truth, of course, is that you didn't cause the abuse; it's not your fault.

The truth lifts us from the burdens of our past and frees us from the anxieties of our future. For example, while it's true that you didn't cause the abuse to happen, you're responsible for the mental processes that perpetuate the suffering and limitations you experience today. That truth doesn't necessarily feel good, but the truth doesn't carry the weightiness of the illusion.

The effort of releasing the bonds with your painful past is why I love the opening quote by Lily Tomlin and chose it for this chapter: *"Forgiveness is giving up all hope of a better past."* Demanding that the past be different is an emotional trap that binds you to its history. You can hear your ego prodding you, *"That abuse should never have happened to me."* Or *"My life should have followed a different path."* Or *"I wish I grew up in a home with two loving parents."* You can feel the weight of those statements.

Forgiveness isn't about absolving the other person of the offense; it's not about Sara forgiving her uncle for his abuse. It's not about forgetting, approving, or denying what occurred in your past. Nor does it mean appeasement and then opening yourself up to being hurt again. Your forgiveness isn't for the abuser; it's for you. It's the gift you give yourself in terms of self-care and freedom. Your forgiveness allows you to live according to *your* values, which is made possible by surrendering to reality.

It Couldn't Have Happened Any Other Way

Marsha M. Linehan is an American psychologist and the creator of Dialectical Behavior Therapy, a type of psychotherapy designed for under-controlled people that combines behavioral science with concepts such as acceptance and mindfulness. Dr. Linehan notes that the enduring stigma of mental illness (in this context, trauma) teaches people to think of themselves as victims, snuffing out the one thing that can motivate them to find treatment: hope. In *Building a Life Worth Living*, Linehan shares how "you can build a life experienced as worth living" by finding mindful ways of accepting yourself and managing your emotions.[46]

Linehan uses the metaphor of an accident at an intersection. A drunk driver is careening down a road toward a crossing at the bottom of the hill. At that very same time, a 12-year-old boy on his bike is crossing that intersection. The drunk driver, not paying attention that the light has changed to red, hits the boy on the bike. Linehan's point is that the laws of physics required that what happened to that 12-year-old boy at that moment in time did indeed happen; it could not have unfolded any other way. By extension, everything in our lives happened because it could not have happened any other way. Sure, you can prefer that reality be different than it is, that the boy not have gotten hit. However, we're still faced with reality. This gives us a choice: we can

---

[46] Linehan, Marsha M. (January 7, 2020). *Building a Life Worth Living: A Memoir*. Random House. Retrieved from https://www.amazon.com/Building-Life-Worth-Living-Memoir/dp/0812994612/ref=tmm_hrd_swatch_0?_encoding=UTF8&qid=1652878648&sr=8-4

live as a victim of the past, or we can accept its truth, forgive it, and live in the present.

Carlos came to see me for sex therapy. He struggled with his sexuality and feelings of sexual inadequacies. He shared with me that he had been sexually assaulted when he was 12 years old by a priest while serving as an altar boy. In a state of exacerbation, Carlos exclaimed, *"I just wish I could get over this, but the past haunts me."*

"Carlos, first, I hate that this happened to you. I see the pain behind your eyes. I hear you say that you want to get past this, and you believe the thought that the past haunts you. I know that it seems like the past haunts you, Carlos. It feels like it blinds you, and you can't escape it. Can I share a story with you?" I asked.

"Yes, of course," he replied.

"Two Buddhist monks are walking down a path after a rainfall. As they walk along, they encounter a woman standing in front of an overflowing stream that has blocked the path. The older monk picks up the woman, carries her across the stream, and puts her down, whereby she and the two monks continue on their separate journeys. After a few miles, the younger monk says to the elder, 'We took a vow not to touch women, yet you carried that woman across the stream.' The older monk paused and replied, 'I put that woman down miles ago. Who's carrying her now?'"

I go on, *"Carlos, the past can't haunt you. It's over there; it's not here. However, you can haunt the past by rehearsing the memory without extracting meaning. Healing begins by finding meaning in your history while thriving in the present where you are free of the abuse."* I then asked, *"Carlos, you've told me that the priest assaulted you twice, is that correct?"*

"Yes," he affirmed.

I asked, *"And how many times have you thought about the abuse over these past decades? Thousands of times, right? Can you see where all of the abuse is happening? I mean, twice is already tragic, but the abuse isn't happening now and hasn't happened since except in your mind. Here's why Byron Katie observed, 'Reality is always kinder than your thoughts.' Can you see how reality—this moment in which you and I find ourselves where no abuse is happening—is way kinder?"*

Carlos isn't unique, of course. Years ago, I attended a retreat for male survivors of sexual abuse. And of course, if you know me, I can't just stop being a therapist—it's in my blood! So, while I was there for my learning and development, I was also observing the other men and listening. I found I could easily categorize these men into two groups: high-functioning survivors and those who were less functioning. I saw that the men who struggled the most were those who attributed current struggles to their past abuse.

The men functioning well, and I included myself in that group, also shared their stories. Yet the pattern that emerged was no one linked current life experiences, including struggles, to our past abuse. We each spoke of recognizing and accepting that we were grown men with responsibilities. We weren't going to have our abusers maintain any power over us. We get to make choices today and live a life of our own agency rather than blame any misfortunes on an abused past. This was foundational for us being able to move forward.

Growing Beyond the Trauma

In times of stress, crisis, or trauma, people like Sara and Carlos often ask after the incident or experience, *"What good can come of this?"* Sometimes the experience is so severe that the answer might be, *"No good can ever come from this."*

Yet at some point, we can reflect on the consequences. Almost always those reflections will include comforting and discomforting thoughts. Therapists refer to it as *post-traumatic growth (PTG)*, a theory that explains the positive transformation following trauma that most experience. It was developed by psychologists Richard Tedeschi and Lawrence Calhoun in the mid-1990s and held that people who endure psychological struggles following adversity often experience positive growth afterward.[47]

Throughout history, we have found that negative experiences can stimulate positive change, such as recognizing your strength, the emergence of new possibilities, enhanced or renewed relationships, a greater appreciation for life, and spiritual growth. Famed psychiatrist and Holocaust survivor Victor Frankl wrote, "When we are no longer able to change a situation, we are challenged to change ourselves." Traumatic events aren't the end of the road. Instead, the trauma can catapult people towards positive action in their lives.

The research on PTG allows you to benefit from what's been discovered to work for those who've recovered after a traumatic experience. With these tools, you can rewrite the trauma narrative and avoid falling prey to the trappings of the ego's investment in victimhood.

PTG highlights valuable tools and lessons that enable this transformation and prove that, despite the misery, we still can expect to grow in beneficial ways in its aftermath through education, emotional regulation, disclosure, narrative development, and service. As I define each, think of your situation and how you can apply these five exercises towards PTG to support your growth and strengthen your ability to unshackle yourself from your past.

Education

Knowledge is the first and most important tool. As you move through trauma to growth, you begin by learning and understanding the truth about the trauma and why it happened. Ask yourself, *"What is there for me to learn here?"*

---

[47] Tedeschei, Richard G. (July–August, 2020). *Growth After Trauma*. Harvard Business Review. Retrieved from https://hbr.org/2020/07/growth-after-trauma.

The initial element in Dr. Ellis' Rational Emotive Behavior Therapy helps address that question. The "rational" part of the therapy is knowledge, which corrects dysfunctional reasonings and frees you from your assumptions and biases. Ultimately, education can help you manage your emotions and build better relationships. This is why rational thinking and gaining knowledge is the first step. It opens your mind to forgiving, accepting yourself and what happened, learning from it, and living in the present.

Emotional Regulation

You can regulate your emotions directly by observing and engaging them as they are experienced. However, you must first be in the right frame of mind and stay grounded and present, open and available. The frame of mind you're looking for is the awareness that you can tolerate difficult emotions. Just simply affirming that you're capable is exceedingly powerful.

Shane realized this firsthand. He, like Carlos, attributed his anxiety about sex to his trauma history. He described being humiliated, embarrassed, and ridiculed while being sexually assaulted by his older sister. Now in his late 20s, he's finally sought help to address his compulsive pursuit of perfectionism, believing that that would eliminate any sense of sexual inadequacy. During our work together, Shane was encouraged to ask himself a powerful question, *"Can I experience more awkwardness and anxiety and still survive if it means that I get to have more of what I say I want?"* His answer was always, *"Yes."* Consequently, he was better able to self-regulate without running from discomfort. He perceived the discomfort as an opportunity for growth.

Disclosure

Divulging what happened is the next stage in the process. In this stage, you openly share your trauma story and what you've contended with in its aftermath. Your ability to disclose and explain those things helps you make sense of your trauma and turn debilitating thoughts into more-productive reflections. This is particularly true if you've never told your story before. Moreover, disclosure is an expression of vulnerability, a skill we've discussed throughout this book to cultivate more meaningful and fulfilling relationships.

Narrative Development

What do you want your legacy to be now that you've survived your abuse? What is the story you want people to say about you? Narrative development creates an accurate and honest chronicle about the trauma and your life afterward. Your goal is to unearth the truth, accept what happened in your life, and describe how your life will now be with your current knowledge. This is where you are now consciously shifting from a trauma narrative to a healing narrative. This shift in narrative allows you to take charge by defining your trauma; your trauma no longer defines you. Much of what was discussed in the prior sections of this chapter can help inform your answers to the questions that opened this section.

Service

Evidence shows that doing something to serve others can also benefit your mental health and wellbeing. People do better in the aftermath of trauma if they find work that helps others. It can reduce stress and improve mood, self-esteem, and happiness. It can also increase your knowledge and prove to yourself that you're shedding the victimhood mindset.

There are many ways to help others as part of your everyday life. Good deeds needn't take much time or cost a lot. This service element brings us back to RO DBT and the feeling of being part of a tribe or member of a community. When you feel part of a community, there's greater resiliency for every group member because they're standing together and supporting each other in ways seen and unseen, felt and unfelt. It's similar to a stand of trees that withstand gale-force winds that would otherwise break a single tree standing alone. There's strength in numbers.

Getting Back to the Goal

I'll often ask my patients, *"Who is made right by your continued struggle with yourself and fear and avoidance of sex?"* They'll generally respond with, *"No one. No one is made right."* Under closer scrutiny, my patients realize that those who stole their joy of sexual pleasure are made right when the abused maintain their unrelenting internal battle. By that, I mean the abuser stole their joy, believing it was theirs to take. The abuser is made right when we don't reclaim our happiness.

Suppose you're sexually traumatized and experience an unsatisfying or problematic sex life because you're continuing to relive the past or fear the future. This only benefits your abuser and anyone else in your life who's led you to believe that sex is wrong or evil. By living with a victimhood mindset, all those people are made right. Let's make them wrong!

To paraphrase George Herbert, a 16th-century poet, "The best revenge is a well-lived life." If so, reclaiming your sexuality is the best revenge. Take heed, though, that recapturing your sexual self and sexual narrative must be because you want something better for yourself. It can't be solely because your partner is dissatisfied with the frequency or quality of *their* sex life. It can't be because you're afraid your partner will leave you or worry that you'll be alone forever if you don't get your shit together.

Ultimately, your progress toward making nice with naughty requires examining your sexual motivations. Sexual motivations are best when they move you in the direction you want to go with your sexual self and intimate relationships. Staci Haines, author of *Healing Sex: A Mind-Body Approach to Healing Sexual Trauma,* provides several examples of healthy motivations for sexual healing.[48] Here are just a few. There's space below for you to express your healthy motivations for sexual healing.

- *"I want to heal the shame that runs my sex life so that I feel relaxed and excited during sex."*
- *"I want to enjoy touching myself."*
- *"I want to have sex in the ways I am interested in. I want to be more courageous sexually."*
- *"I want to have sex and intimacy at the same time."*

Reclaiming your joy means becoming intrinsically motivated to engage in this effort of making nice with naughty. It cannot be for your partner. It's for you, wanting to heal the shame that runs your sex life, that ruins your sex life. You want to feel relaxed. You want to feel excited during sex. You want to enjoy touching yourself. You want to have sex in ways that you're interested in. Your motivation comes from realizing that you're missing something you have every right to experience.

Staci Haines' concept of healthy motivations for sexual healing parallels the exercise I discussed in Chapter 4: "What is Your Desire Narrative?" There I introduced an approach called Solution-Focused Brief Therapy (SFBT), a solution-oriented, goal-directed therapy

---

[48] Haines, Staci (September 1, 2007). *Healing Sex: A Mind-Body Approach to Healing Sexual Trauma.* Retrieved from https://www.amazon.com/Healing-Sex-Mind-Body-Approach-Sexual/dp/1573442933/ref=sr_1_1?crid=10Y9I1O3OD2SP&keywords=Healing+Sex%3A+A+Mind-Body+Approach+to+Healing+Sexual+Trauma&qid=1652919933&sprefix=healing+sex+a+mind-body+approach+to+healing+sexual+trauma%2Caps%2C303&sr=8-1

focused on possibilities and strengths rather than problems, weaknesses, or deficits.

Ask yourself what can help you move from a victimhood mindset to a desire narrative of what you long for in your sexual and intimate relationships. What do you wish for; what is your goal? As I go through this exercise with Sara, think of your desire narrative and those things that are comfortable for you to share and experience with your partner.

After going through the ABCs of Sara's thoughts and feelings with her about not being able to enjoy herself sexually, I focus her attention on her goal of greater intimacy with her partner and being more comfortable in engaging in sex. I asked Sara to begin framing her desire narrative by describing what living her goal would look and feel like. *"How do you want to be with your partner, Sara? What would you want your partner to know that's goal-related for you?"*

While Sara responds with her desire narrative, reflect on what yours would be:

- *"I would be less distressed by my thoughts."*
- *"I'd like to experiment with having sex in places other than in bed."*
- *"I want him to talk to me while we're making love so I can hear his voice and know it's him, especially in the dark."*
- *"I want to have sex outside the house, like in a hotel, just for the night."*

After discussing her vision, Sara and I set out to identify alternative beliefs that support these outcomes. *"Sara, let's suppose that you had all of these things. You've identified a number of desires. Now, let's go upstream. What thoughts would you be having that would naturally lead to these desires?"*

Sara, building on our prior sessions, aims for more flexible, adaptive responses: *"While it's my preference to not have intrusive thoughts, the truth is that I can just notice them rather than get caught up in them. I can bring myself back to this moment where there's nothing wrong."* She goes on to say,

"Being awkward isn't the end of the world. I'm breaking no law in experimenting sexually with Brian. I'm willing to feel awkward if it means having more of what I want."

Finally, she adds, *"It's better for me to speak up and tell Brian what I want from him to help me better enjoy myself. He's responsible for his reaction to my requests. While I would prefer him to accommodate me, there's no rule that he must. He's a separate person and likely has preferences of his own. There's room for negotiation."*

Sara intuits that her transition from victim to victorious on her journey towards making nice with naughty requires a shift in how she thinks about her abuse history. Her transition reflects psychological flexibility whereby she retains agency over her sexuality. Moreover, Sara embraces and prioritizes her own sexual motivations for making positive changes in how she thinks. She's cultivated acceptance around her abuse history having "[given] up all hope for a better past."

FORGIVENESS EXERCISE

As with every other chapter in this book, this chapter aims to help you make nice with naughty and reclaim your enjoyment of sexual pleasure and fulfillment as a sexual being. Forgiveness is an essential part of that reclamation, as is experiencing post-traumatic growth. Recall, however, that forgiveness isn't an act in the service of the abuser. Instead, forgiveness is an act of self-love that releases the chains that bind you to a painful past. With those shackles broken and fallen away, you're free to pursue your goals.

To that end, Dr. Thomas Lynch uses an exercise in RO DBT that I also use in my practice called HEART: identify the past **H**urt; locate your **E**dge that's keeping you stuck in the past; **A**cknowledge that forgiveness is a choice; **R**eclaim your life by grieving your loss and practicing forgiveness; practice **T**hankfulness and pass it on.[49]

Before beginning this exercise, let's get centered. Sit resting comfortably in your chair with your back relaxed. Bring your attention to your breathing. Inhaling. Exhaling. You'll likely find your feelings shifting toward a calmer state. Moreover, just as eyebrow raises release positive hormones, deep breathing has the effect of calming your nerves and reducing your anxiety. From this improved state, you'll find yourself more flexible and open to this exercise.

Identify the Past Hurt

Engaging with the painful event is the first step toward forgiveness. What past grievance, injury, abuse, or event keeps you from experiencing an enjoyable and fulfilling sex life? What past event or experience do you want to avoid, pretend never happened, or try to forget? Call it out now.

---

[49] Lynch (n 1), pp 506–515.

"My painful event occurred when…"

Locate Your Edge

To let go of a past grievance or injury, you must first find your edge that keeps you holding on to the abuse and keeps you stuck in the past. This edge is where self-growth actually occurs. It's that point where you're inclined to turn away from it because it's uncomfortable, awkward, or anxiety-provoking. Your edge may be something in your sexual life that you don't want to think about or admit to. Ask yourself: Who are you hurting or helping by holding onto this pain? What do you think keeps you from letting go of your traumatic thoughts? What is it that you're afraid would happen if you were to forgive? Define your edge here.

"My edge that keeps me stuck in the past is…"

Acknowledge that Forgiveness Is a Choice

Forgiveness is a choice that only you can make. It is ultimately your decision. Keep in mind that not deciding is still making a choice. What is it that you want to come to accept about your past? You might begin with the following and conclude with your acknowledgment:

> *"I've come to accept that…*
>
> *Despite my preference for the contrary, it had to happen as it did. There's no other way that it could have unfolded. And, I survived it."*

Reclaim Your Life

Sexual trauma, in particular, can shake your trust in the world and in humanity. To forgive and reclaim your life, you must first grieve the loss of your expectations and beliefs about your sexual abuse. Grieving the abuse means allowing yourself to feel the sadness or disappointment associated with it and then releasing the sadness instead of holding it inside as despair and hopelessness. Sadness is a healthy negative emotion and helps you recognize that you cannot control the world. In the space below, identify how you want to show up as a sexual person free from the chains that bound you to the past.

> *"I want to experience greater intimacy and sexuality in my relationships by…"*

Practice Thankfulness

Cultivating gratitude shifts the victimhood mindset. Practice being thankful for having the resources that guided you to this point in your life. You being here isn't by accident. You co-created this moment. You made decisions that brought you here. For example, you are alive, you have a roof over your head, you have your health, you are learning new skills and having new experiences every day. Who and what are you thankful for?

Be thankful when an opportunity for forgiveness arises. Let's take a look at the root of forgiveness. Forgiveness literally means to *give* in the way you did *before* the transgression. Again, we're not necessarily talking about your relationship with your abuser. Often one's abuser doesn't deserve that kind of forgiveness. Rather, we're talking about how you treat yourself. Every child intuitively knows how to play, explore, and pursue adventure. Forgiveness in this context is to give to yourself in the way you did before the abuse. When you give to yourself, you're cultivating a context for gratitude.

How does gratitude look for you in the context of your trauma history? What have you learned about yourself as a survivor? See yourself as I see you, capable, competent, complete, whole, and enough.

> *"As a survivor, I learned and grew from my knowledge that..."*
>
> *"By forgiving, I express care for myself by letting go of my useless and non-productive anger, shame, and self-criticism. By forgiving, I allow myself to live according to my values and reclaim my enjoyment of sexual pleasure and fulfillment as a sexual being.*

CHAPTER 10

COMMITTING TO THE VISION

"Commitment is an act, not a word."

— Jean-Paul Sartre

"I had every intention to make nice with naughty, Dr. Tom," Kirk sheepishly offered during a recent session. *"I thought all day about how I wanted to show Elaine that I'm sexually interested in her, but I couldn't get past the critic in my head. I thought about it all day, and the next day, and the next day, and the day after that. I envisioned what I wanted to do but felt frozen when it was time to do something."*

He continued, *"I still hear echoes of my history that make me question my thoughts about sex. I don't feel confident I can enjoy sex without feeling guilty, ashamed, awkward, or embarrassed. The uncertainty is like quicksand. I feel myself sinking and immobilized to do anything."*

"Ah, yes," I said, *"I'm familiar with the quicksand analogy. The more you struggle, the more stuck you feel. In your case, the more your thoughts are focused on fighting anxiety and believing that you must get rid of these feelings FIRST before taking action, the more you fear you'll sink, lose control, and not be able to save yourself."*

"That pretty much sums it up, Doc."

"Kirk, what's the real danger here? Is it the quicksand or the sinking? In other words, is the anxiety dangerous, or is it your struggle with anxiety that's impeding your progress?" I asked.

"I suppose it's the struggle."

"And your ultimate goal is to be free from the quicksand, right?"

"For sure, to be free of the anxiety," Kirk exclaimed after making the connection.

"Right. So, in your scenario, it's assumed that there are no tools to which you have access to pull yourself out of the quicksand; otherwise, you'd have used them, right?"

"Yeah, I wouldn't be here with you if I already had the tools!"

"Makes perfect sense to me," I affirmed. *"So, there are no tools, and the struggle is the danger, not the anxiety. Are you willing to try something different?"* Kirk nodded his approval. *"Okay, good,"* I said, *"Lay flat on the quicksand."*

"What!" Kirk exclaimed incredulously. *"You want me to lay flat on the quicksand?"*

I reiterated, *"Yes, lay flat and don't struggle. Make more contact with the quicksand. In the absence of any struggle, you won't sink, right? You'd be unstuck and able to roll your body toward safety, wouldn't you?"*

I then shared a most important point with him: *"Once you stop struggling, you are actually taking action to get away from the quicksand that is your anxiety. Ironically, when you engage anxiety by taking committed action that aligns with your desire to make nice with naughty, you're that much closer to getting more of what you want. And isn't that why we're here—so you can have more of what you want?"*

Kirk fell prey to the seductive thought that he must be free of the anxiety to show his wife that he's sexually interested in her. He's been ruminating about what he needs to do, but he stalls when the rubber hits the road. That's because he's not taking committed action in the face of his anxiety.

At this point, I challenged Kirk. *"It's your choice, you know? You can communicate your sexual desire to your wife without sinking. All you have to do is trust that you can lie flat, in full contact with the sand so that you can roll toward sexual freedom."*

"No, I can't," Kirk responded, still unconvinced. *"Not yet. Not until I'm over this anxiety. It has to be 100 percent gone. I must be certain and confident in how my attempts will play out. I can't tolerate surprises."*

"Let me propose something," I said. *"Suppose I have one million dollars, and all you have to do to get that million is to, once a day, for a month, communicate to Elaine the simple message that you desire her sexually. Do you think you would be able to do that? Yes or No, no conditions."*

Kirk did some quick math in his head and chuckled as he responded, *"Of course! That's like $30,000 a message!"*

"Well then, it seems it's a choice you're making; it's not the anxiety or your struggle with the anxiety, now is it?" I asked. Crickets, as Kirk pondered the thought that he was willing to co-exist with his feelings of anxiety, that he actually could consider it.

People get caught up in the thought that they have to be free of discomfort, whatever it is, before they feel confident to take action. Just like Kirk, you may have found yourself struggling with taking action toward making nice with naughty, yet you're taking some risks to get there. You've taken a significant step in making it to the end of the book with me, bringing you that much closer to making your desire a reality. We're going to cinch it in this chapter as you continue your commitment to your vision.

Recapping Our Journey

Look how far you've come! You read the material and may have even seen yourself in some of my stories. You participated in the exercises found in each chapter and may have implemented a few of the strategies. You turned down the dial on your OC temperament and turned up the dial on your making nice with naughty. I'll wait while you pat yourself on the back. I mean it. Take a moment and reward yourself.

You've now acquired the mindset and self-reinforcing skill sets needed to rationalize, challenge, and change the maladaptive thinking that fuels your anxieties and fears. Let's review the key insights shared in each chapter that have aided you in your journey toward making nice with naughty.

Chapter 1 introduced you to the four key traits of an overcontrolled temperament and the high cost of having too much self-control. I explained how you'd been both biologically programmed to lean overcontrolled and socialized within a family and culture that privileges many characteristics of the OC temperament. Moreover, I underscored how the OCs' intolerance of uncertainty drives much of their behavior in adaptive and maladaptive ways.

Chapter 2 linked your OC thoughts and actions—although valuable in other avenues of your life—to your struggles with sexuality and intimacy in your relationships. I explained how the same admirable qualities that have served you well throughout your life at the same time might pose challenges for you in the bedroom and in establishing and maintaining long-term, intimate relationships.

Chapter 3 buttressed you with the notion that the little voice inside your head—that narrator of your life—isn't really *you*. You came to the awareness that *you* are not your experience; instead, *you* are that who *observes* your experience. And you now know that if there's any hope of making nice with naughty, you need to start embracing the real *you* from this higher perspective.

In ***Chapter 4***, you discovered that reigniting desire requires (1) **fuel**, the small, everyday contributions to the relationship, including those unexpected, spontaneous ways of being present and proactively engaged, and (2) **oxygen**, the embodied view of yourself as a sexual being deserving of sexual expression and fulfillment that is free of anxiety and fear.

Chapter 5 brought a greater realization of how the OC trait of a neutral face to veil feelings of vulnerability or conceal your thoughts and emotions can work to your advantage in some contexts, such as funerals or business meetings, yet can be misconstrued as threatening, stand-offish, and aloof when it comes to intimate relationships. You learned why an amiable countenance and intentional eyebrow raises, even if "simulated," can activate neuroregulatory systems that trigger positive feelings within you, as well as positive emotions within your partner.

In *Chapter 6*, I applied the concept of values to the context of making nice with naughty to help you clarify what's important to you vis-à-vis your sexual behavior. Your values serve as guideposts for living an authentic life. Therefore, I invited you to examine whether your sexual and intimate behaviors reflect your values. You know now that values are not goals, wants, or needs. Values reflect what's most important to you and what brings meaning and purpose to your life. They are your lighthouse, giving you a focal point for gauging your actions. Values aren't dependent on outcomes or others' behaviors, nor do they conflict with each other.

Chapter 7 provided a framework to help change your relationship with anxiety—to learn to live with it and even draw strength from it by creating an optimum balance that allows you to reclaim your innate sexual self. I facilitated your making friends with your fears, worries, and concerns by helping you distinguish healthy from unhealthy forms of anxiety and separate rational from irrational thoughts. You learned strategies to support your new reasoning by (1) disputing unfounded beliefs and (2) experiencing the positive effect healthier thoughts can have on your sex life and the sex life of your partner.

By this point in the book, I expect you've accepted who you are and know how your OC temperament affects your capacity to make nice with naughty. *Chapter 8* offered a series of mindfulness meditations designed to help turn down the volume on your mind-chatter and bring you closer to the optimum balance you discovered within yourself through the values check and clarification exercises in Chapter 7.

This book wouldn't be complete if I didn't devote a chapter to those who have experienced sexual trauma in their lives and how their experience intersects with the value of making nice with naughty. In *Chapter 9*, you learned why the story we tell ourselves about our trauma is the biggest impediment to finding enjoyment and fulfillment in our sexual life and intimate relationships. You also found that forgiveness is an act of self-love and an essential part of your ability to grow from victim to victorious and reclaim or claim, for the first time in your life, yourself as a sexual being.

Here in *Chapter 10*, you're committing to your vision. In your transformation, I want to ensure that your values are what's guiding you to more sexually satisfying and intimate relationships. I want to have a bit of a reality check between us to ensure that you are not mistaking values for goals or outcomes, which are usually dependent on the intentions or needs of others.

Making Nice with Naughty Isn't the Goal

Making nice with naughty isn't the goal. *"Then why in the f*ck am I reading this book?"* you might ask. Let me explain. The intent of Chapter 6 was to help you clarify your values as to what actions to take when things become uncertain and stressful in your life. Unlike goals or outcomes, values are not destinations. For instance, making nice with naughty is not a goal or a destination; it's your North Star, your value as a sexual being, guiding your movements toward what's important to you in your daily attempts to live an authentic life. You achieve this by identifying the goals pertaining to that value and breaking down those intentions into identifiable, actionable steps. Goals are the initiatives you have total control over and can't be dependent upon another person, such as increasing communication of your sexual desire to your partner, being more open to novel ideas, or being more sensitive to your partner's sexual needs and reactions.

As we learned from Kirk at the top of the chapter, he initially said his goal was for his wife, Elaine, to trust that he was sexually interested in her. Of course, I helped Kirk realize that changing his wife's thoughts and feelings about him weren't goals but outcomes. He didn't have direct control over how Elaine felt or how she thought. My explanation gave Kirk pause as he thought more about his values. Then he landed on what was important in his life and stated, *"Being a sexually interested and expressive husband."*

"Perfect," I responded. *"That value will be your lighthouse and guide you when feeling anxious and uncertain. What's your goal then?"*

Kirk responded with even greater certainty than before. *"My objective now is to communicate my sexual desire for my wife. And through my actions, she'll know I sexually desire her."*

That's the outcome Kirk was hoping for—Elaine not only believing but experiencing his desire for her. By beginning with his values and following his heart, he now has goals toward which he can take committed actions that will build her trust in him.

Let's put this to the test for you. In the **Values Check Exercise** from Chapter 6, you illuminated your values relative to sex and sexuality by answering six questions. Choose one of your values from that exercise that you'd like to take committed action on now. I recommend focusing on one that's sexual, romantic, or intimate in nature. After all, you ultimately want to make nice with naughty, right? You can also use the **Values Clarification Table** at the end of that chapter for thought starters. It contains examples of value statements found in Drs. Lev and McKay's book, *Acceptance and Commitment Therapy for Couples*.[50]

---

[50] Lev and McKay (n 25), p 54.

Is It Workable?

There's a tool in Acceptance and Commitment Therapy (ACT) that helps patients reassess their goals and values by helping them identify how they've been avoiding their anxieties, fears, and pains and then evaluating through their lived experience what that avoidance has cost them.

Through this process, people realize that their control and avoidance strategies haven't worked or have actually been counterproductive, distancing them from their values and most desired intentions. This process, called *Creative Hopelessness*, can help stop unworkable behavior and open the way to new, more workable strategies.[51]

The idea is that people work so hard and try all kinds of strategies to eliminate their discomfort. The question is, how workable is it to constantly focus on getting rid of your discomfort and getting you to the desired outcome? How successful has that been for you relative to what you ultimately want? Letting go of the hope that the strategies will work opens the door to value-oriented behavior and space for something new. The irony is that by developing acceptance of your life situation, you realize that you can never totally rid yourself of your anxiety; you just accept that discomfort is a part of life.

Ultimately, your goals related to making nice with naughty can be broken down into long-term and short-term goals. A long-term goal might be to develop greater acceptance of yourself as a sexual person. A short-term goal might be to ensure you greet and hug your partner the first thing when either you or your partner comes home after a long day at work. Regardless of how you defined the goal, the goal must ultimately be workable. In other words, the goal must be consistent with how you live your life.

---

[51] Ibid, p 82.

In my experience, if you're required to make substantial changes to your lifestyle to take action and meet the goal, you will most likely not take action. To that end, when it comes to your goal, ask yourself the following questions:

- Does the goal fit within my current life situation?
- Do I have total control over achieving the goal?
- Would completing the goal move me in the direction I want to go vis-à-vis making nice with naughty?

Let's return to Kirk's value of being a sexually interested and expressive husband. His stated value can be further broken down into two parts: (1) sexually interested (cognitive) and (2) expressive (behavioral). Therefore, his goals must be achievable and obtainable mentally and physically. The challenge is that Kirk wants to be free of awkwardness and anxiety before taking action. He wants his wife to know he's invested in her, but you can see how *"being free of awkwardness and anxiety"* isn't going to be workable for him and produce the desired outcome. Kirk will need to identify the workable goals, steps, and committed action he can take to live his value of being a more sexually interested and expressive partner to Elaine.

The Recipe

Every cookbook contains logical, step-by-step instructions designed to help you achieve the outcome you're looking for in the kitchen. The best cookbook authors leave little room for interpretation. Instead, they break down the recipe into a series of specific and achievable steps until the culinary masterpiece is achieved. My favorite cookbooks are the ones that also include pictures of the end product. I prefer to know what the dish is supposed to look like when complete. (Can you see my OC peeking through the Peking Duck?)

I've adapted the Values and Goals Worksheet from *ACT on Life, Not on Anger* by psychologists Drs. Georg Eifert, Matthew McKay, and

Making Nice with Naughty

John Forsyth as a recipe card for assisting you in the process of identifying your goals, steps, and committed actions to live your value[52] and help you achieve the outcome you're looking for in the bedroom (or kitchen).

Once you've identified your value, list the goals that will enable you to live that value. Make sure they are workable goals (i.e., they can easily be made a part of your life; you have total control in achieving each goal; the goals move you in the direction you want). The next part of the recipe is to break each goal down into smaller, logical steps. If the order doesn't matter, start with the easiest step.

When confronted by their anxieties and fears, many believe they must conquer those feelings, break through the anxiety, and rid themselves of their distressing thoughts. Instead, you can simply walk around the obstacle or climb over it. You don't have to vanquish the anxious thoughts and uncertain feelings. You can transform them into something adaptive that can co-exist with your value of making nice with naughty.

In the table below, declare your naughty value, your naughty goals, and the sexy recipe steps you'll take to achieve your goals. Next, list the obstacle(s) you believe you'll encounter to take each step on your list. How will the step(s) you take in the service of your values be received by your partner? Once you've listed your steps and the obstacles you might encounter, identify the committed action or actions you'll need to take to walk around the obstacle or climb over it and accomplish that step.

---

[52] Eifert, George H. & McKay, Matthew & Forsyth, John P. (March 3, 2006). *ACT on Life Not on Anger: The New Acceptance and Commitment Therapy Guide to Problem Anger*. New Harbinger Publications. Retrieved from, https://www.amazon.com/ACT-Life-Not-Anger-Acceptance/dp/1572244402/ref=sr_1_1?crid=3TTMJ3QM1EMS3&keywords=ACT+on+Life%2C+Not+on+Anger&qid=1657545115&sprefix=act+on+life%2C+not+on+anger+%2Caps%2C108&sr=8-1

During our session, Kirk filled in the worksheet based on his value of being a sexually interested and expressive husband to Elaine. We used this exercise to deconstruct his value to include his goal statement, steps to achieve his goal, the obstacles he believed will be there, and the committed actions he was prepared to take to circumvent each obstacle. Most importantly, he listed when he would take the steps and committed actions to achieve his goal.

Making Nice with Naughty Goals Worksheet

My Naughty Value: To be a more sexually interested and expressive husband					
Naughty Goal:	**Sexy Recipe Steps**	**Obstacles**	**Committed Actions**	**When?**
Communicate to my wife my sexual desire for her.	Be open to my partner's bids for sex.	Feeling anxious for not being mentally and physically ready.	View my partner's bid as an opportunity to play and not a need to perform.	Any time my partner is interested in sex.
	Text my desire for my partner.	My message appearing out of the blue and embarrassing myself. Seeming insincere.	Send a silly text and embarrass myself on purpose anyway.	At least twice a week.
	Make the first move.	She may not be interested and say no. She will be interested and I freeze up.	Embrace your perfectionism and live with it. Try new things and be kind to the part of me that isn't perfect.	Whenever the mood strikes me. Look for her tell-tale signs.

"Do Or Do Not; There Is No Try"

After Kirk filled in his worksheet, he looked over the committed actions column with a bit of nervousness. *"I mean, I feel like I'm trying.*

Making Nice with Naughty

Filling out this table is proof I'm trying," Kirk remarked as he fidgeted on the couch. I grabbed a tissue from its box and placed it on the arm of the sofa next to him.

"Kirk, I want you to try to pick up the tissue."

Kirk's hand moved toward the tissue and clinched the paper with his index finger and thumb, raising it off the couch. *"Kirk, I didn't say pick up the tissue."* Kirk reactively put the tissue back on the arm of the sofa. *"I said* try *to pick up the tissue."* He motioned toward the tissue, picking it up once again. *"No, Kirk, you're picking up the tissue; I said* try *to pick it up."*

A smile came across Kirk's face as his gaze shifted from looking at the tissue to meeting my eyes. *"I get it now. I'm either picking up the tissue, or I'm not. There's no trying."*

"Precisely! I believe Yoda said it best, 'Do, or do not. There is no try.' What Yoda taught young Luke was a simple lesson in commitment and the power in giving something our all, and not just giving it a try. Trying doesn't accomplish much. You either decide that you can and do it or decide to quit. When you said you would do it for a million dollars, you told me you could do it if you decided.

"When you picked up the tissue, you took committed action. The doing is the proof of the wanting. When someone says that they want to lose weight, what's the proof? Exercising and eating fewer calories. When someone says they want to write a book, what's the evidence that they want to?"

Kirk responded, *"Setting time and putting pen to paper."*

"You bet. Regardless of how you feel, right? I mean, if you tell me that you want to lose weight, yet you're not exercising or eating fewer calories, the evidence suggests that you want something other than to lose weight."

There's a therapeutic technique called "paradoxical intervention" where therapists direct their patients to continue undesired behavior and even increase it to prove to their patients have voluntary control over the behavior. In the context of making nice with naughty, if you're afraid to sound foolish, as an example, and the fear of sounding foolish prevents you from taking action, or the fear of not being sexually perfect holds you back, then be intentional about sounding foolish or being imperfect.

The whole idea of needing to be the perfect husband versus a good enough husband comes down to acceptance. Elaine just wants evidence that Kirk is trying. The evidence is necessary for her to trust that he's interested in her sexually. Trying without any evidence is the royal road to your partner feeling resentful. Your partner hears, *"I'm trying,"* but there's no proof. Taking committed actions such as the ones Kirk has specified in the worksheet above or the committed actions you've listed in your chart is evidence that you are committing to the vision.

Let me add one more thing here. You can supercharge your committed action by soliciting the support of others. Accountability is a well-regarded fertilizer for behavior change. Moreover, OC people respond well to being held accountable. This step, however, requires vulnerability. In essence, you're admitting to someone that you're less than perfect. At the same time, your disclosure and commitment to the other that you want to move in a certain direction provides the accountability you may need to get the outcome you want. People perform better when they know someone else is observing their behavior. Share your values, goals, and commitment with your partner and gain their support by having them help hold you accountable.

Committing to the Vision

Despite all the effort you put into breaking down your goals and identifying the practical steps moving forward, progress isn't always a straight line. Indeed, progress is affected by obstacles that get in the way, such as the ones you've noted above. As an OC, you've most likely developed many contingency plans over the course of your life. You have a history of getting what you want through hard work and persistence. However, as this book has highlighted throughout, learning to make nice with naughty involves domains of your life where the same rules tend not to apply.

In Chapter 7, I applied the analogy of holding onto the steering wheel of a car that's out of alignment to holding onto the wheel of your relationship to keep you and your partner from driving off into a ditch. Committed actions are the adjustments you make with the wheel to move your car in the right direction. Now, the fatalistic mindset would say, *"Fuck it. I have no control over this car. I'm just going to crash into the pole. There's nothing I can do about it,"* which we saw initially with Kirk. Of course, you don't do that, do you? You take committed action, grab the wheel and turn the car back in the direction you want to go because you know the results if you don't.

In helping Kirk commit to his vision, I shared the accountability strategy with him and explained how the most powerful committed action I've seen my patients employ when making nice with naughty was by sharing their internal struggles with their partner. To that end, I explained how accountability can boost his actions and help him achieve his goal sooner with Elaine. I encouraged him to lay flat on the quicksand of anxiety and not struggle with it but to embrace it by texting his wife the next time he thought about her sexually and share that he was desirous of her but experiencing anxious feelings.

During Kirk's follow-up appointment, he described how the fear of vulnerability became the primary obstacle once he introduced the accountability strategy into the equation. Nevertheless, Kirk took my advice, and he and his wife discussed this dynamic one evening while they sat on the deck of their lake house. Ironically, Kirk found that simply talking about opening up in that vulnerable way made him feel closer to Elaine. Moreover, she demonstrated further that she could be trusted to hold Kirk's vulnerability. She realized that what was underneath Kirk's anxiety was his desperation to be the husband that she wanted—to be the kind of sexual partner that would please her.

Yet sexual perfectionism got in the way. Kirk felt confident that his wife wanted a perfect husband, and those feelings were just fanned by the societal pressure around masculinity and what it means to be a sexual man.

As our work progressed, Kirk continued to apply the cognitive strategies I shared with you in the previous chapters (drawn from Ellis' Rational Emotive Behavior Therapy and its ABC method, Acceptance and Commitment Therapy, and Radically Open Dialectical Behavior Therapy) to cultivate psychological flexibility. In addition, Kirk and I looked at the value of aiming for being "good enough" rather than perfect. In his case, he was to aim at being a "good enough lover" and a "good enough husband." These values became his proverbial North Star that he used to determine whether his behavior was moving him in the right direction. Moreover, Kirk and I affirmed that everything he wants lies just on the other side of comfort. He will learn what it means to be good enough only by taking committed action. In short, he will only learn through doing!

The major turning point for Kirk was when he finally realized that he could make room for all of the internal obstacles on his journey toward making nice with naughty. We often don't consider "acceptance" a committed action, but it is. Acceptance is a very active process, and Kirk experienced it. He understood that his drive to maintain emotional control, where the focus was on getting rid of discomfort in whatever flavor it came in, led him away from what he said he wanted.

Moreover, Kirk eventually saw the costs to him and his relationship for believing that he had to get rid of discomfort first. It was a strategy that wasn't working for him, his wife, or their relationship. However, acceptance was the doorway he could enter to arrive at a new place.

"Where Do You Want to Go?"

When you got into my taxi, I asked you this question at the end of Chapter 1. You knew deep down that your sex life wasn't moving you in the direction you wanted to go. You accepted that the only reality we would be driving toward was not where you came from but where you want to go to find that lasting, meaningful, intimate relationship that's eluded you.

Perhaps you've learned for the first time that an overcontrolled temperament is a definable thing and is most likely associated with sexual suppression and inhibited sexual satisfaction. You wanted to do something about it and discovered that you can. You stayed with me and now have the open mindset and skill set to move your sex life in the direction you want to go and be the sexual person you deserve.

With heartfelt courage, you've accepted yourself as you are. Moreover, you'll allow yourself to be vulnerable to experience loving connections with your partner and the intimacy you desire. I'm not going to say you'll never have sexual challenges again. But how you navigate unexpected situations will now become more flexible, more fluid, and more rewarding.

My hope for you is that the information, stories, and methodologies I shared during our time together will continue to help you identify and overcome the obstacles that keep you from expressing and finding enjoyment in your sexuality. I wish you a healthy and happy life in your quest to make nice with naughty.

ABOUT THE AUTHOR

Thomas L. Murray, Jr., Ph.D., LMFT (FL, OR, NC, & PA), LCMHCS (NC) is a forensic sexologist and award-winning sex and relationship therapist. He holds certifications through the American Association of Sex Educators, Counselors, and Therapists as a therapist and supervisor. In addition, Dr. Murray is board certified as a forensic mental health evaluator, sex offender treatment provider, and child custody evaluator.

Dr. Murray has been a sought-after speaker, lecturer, and presenter at local, state, and national conferences on topics related to sexuality, social justice, psychopharmacology, clinical effectiveness and ethics, sex therapy and couples' therapy. His commentary has appeared in various online mediums, including *Guardian*, *Huffington Post*, *Daily Mail*, *BBC Online*, and *Fatherly*, as well on various podcasts, including *ShrinkRap Radio*, *Cheating on Fear*, and *Practice of Being Seen*. He's held faculty positions at the Modern Sex Therapy Institute, Adler University, Northwestern University, and Wake Forest University's Department of Psychiatry and Behavioral Medicine, among others.

Dr. Murray earned a Ph.D. in Couple and Family Counseling from the top-ranked Department of Counselor Education at the University of Florida. Currently, he owns and directs A Path to Wellness Integrative Psychiatry in Greensboro, NC, USA. Visit him at www.drtommurray.com or www.apathtowellness.com.

REFERENCES

Albert Ellis Institute. *About Albert Ellis, Ph.D.* Retrieved from https://albertellis.org/about-albert-ellis-phd/.

Aronson, E., Willerman, B., & Floyd, J. (1966). *The Effect of a Pratfall on Increasing Interpersonal Attractiveness. Psychonomic Science, 4*(6). Retrieved from https://psycnet.apa.org/record/1966-05356-001.

Butler EA, Egloff B, Wilhelm FH, Smith NC, Erickson EA, Gross JJ. (March 3, 2003), *The Social Consequences of Expressive Suppression.* Emotion Journal.10.1037/1528–3542.3.1.48. PMID: 12899316. Retrieved from https://pubmed.ncbi.nlm.nih.gov/12899316/.

Chapman, Gary (January 1, 2015). *The 5 Love Languages: The Secret to Love that Lasts.* Northfield Publishing Company. Retrieved from https://www.amazon.com/Love-Languages-Secret-that-Lasts/dp/080241270X/ref=sr_1_1?crid=3UIX2WIMM41JJ&keywords=The+Five+Love+Languages&qid=1642625766&sprefix=the+five+love+languages%2Caps%2C108&sr=8-1

Eifert, George H. & McKay, Matthew & Forsyth, John P. (March 3, 2006). *ACT on Life Not on Anger: The New Acceptance and Commitment Therapy Guide to Problem Anger.* New Harbinger Publications. Retrieved from, https://www.amazon.com/ACT-Life-Not-Anger-Acceptance/dp/1572244402/ref=sr_1_1?crid=3TTMJ3QM1EMS3&keywords=ACT+on+Life%2C+Not+on+Anger&qid=1657545115&sprefix=act+on+life%2C+not+on+anger+%2Caps%2C108&sr=8-1

Fraser, Cheryl Ph.D. (January 2, 2019). *Buddha's Bedroom: The Mindful Loving Path to Sexual Passion and Lifelong Intimacy.* Reveal Press. Retrieved from https://www.amazon.com/Buddhas-Bedroom-Mindful-Lifelong-Intimacy/dp/1684031184.

Gabay, Rahav & Hameiri, Boaz & Rubel-Lifschitz, Tammy & Nadler, Arie (2020). *The Tendency for Interpersonal Victimhood: The Personality Construct and its Consequences.* Personality and Individual Differences, Volume 165. Retrieved from https://doi.org/10.1016/j.paid.2020.110134.

Goodman, Katie (August 1, 2008). *Improvisation for the Spirit: Live a More Creative, Spontaneous, and Courageous Life Using the Tools of Improv Comedy.* Sourcebooks. Retrieved from https://www.amazon.com/Improvisation-Spirit-Creative-Spontaneous-Courageous/dp/1402211910/ref=tmm_pap_swatch_0?_encoding=UTF8&qid=1640366625&sr=8-1

Haines, Staci (May 28, 1999). *The Survivor's Guide to Sex: How to Have an Empowered Sex Life After Child Sexual Abuse.* Cleis Press. Retrieved from https://www.amazon.com/Survivors-Guide-Sex-Empowered-Sexual/dp/1573440795/ref=sr_1_1?crid=ZUI9K3FGPN1R&keywords=the+survivors+guide+to+sex&qid=1656503618&sprefix=the+survivor+s+guide+to+sex%2Caps%2C202&sr=8-1.

Haines, Staci (September 1, 2007). *Healing Sex: A Mind-Body Approach to Healing Sexual Trauma.* Retrieved from https://www.amazon.com/Healing-Sex-Mind-Body-Approach-Sexual/dp/1573442933/ref=sr_1_1?crid=10Y9I1O3OD2SP&keywords=Healing+Sex%3A+A+Mind-Body+Approach+to+Healing+Sexual+Trauma&qid=1652919933&sprefix=healing+sex+a+mind-body+approach+to+healing+sexual+trauma%2Caps%2C303&sr=8-1.

Katie, Byron (December 7, 2021). *Loving What Is: Four Questions That Can Change Your Life.* Harmony Books. Retrieved from https://www.amazon.com/Loving-What-Revised-Questions-Change/dp/0593234510/ref=sr_1_1?crid=26U7G57QBSKPW&

dchild=1&keywords=loving+what+is+revised+edition&qid=1634653945&sprefix=loving+what+is+revised+%2Caps%2C250&sr=8-1&asin=0593234510&revisionId=&format=4&depth=1

Katie, Byron & Katz, Michael (November 28, 2006). *I Need Your Love – Is That True?: How to Stop Seeking Love, Approval, and Appreciation and Start Finding Them Instead.* Harmony Publishing. Retrieved from https://www.amazon.com/Need-Your-Love-Approval-Appreciation/dp/0307345300/ref=asc_df_0307345300/?tag=hyprod-20&linkCode=df0&hvadid=312674808447&hvpos=&hvnetw=g&hvrand=8654632277138145350&hvpone=&hvptwo=&hvqmt=&hvdev=c&hvdvcmdl=&hvlocint=&hvlocphy=9010811&hvtargid=pla-489337318527&psc=1.

Katie, Byron & Mitchell, Stephen (December 7, 2021). *Loving What Is. Revised Edition: Four Questions That Can Change Your Life.* Harmony Publishing. Retrieved from https://www.amazon.com/Loving-What-Revised-Questions-Change/dp/0593234510/ref=asc_df_0593234510/?tag=hyprod-20&linkCode=df0&hvadid=509494905560&hvpos=&hvnetw=g&hvrand=13803923548720416439&hvpone=&hvptwo=&hvqmt=&hvdev=c&hvdvcmdl=&hvlocint=&hvlocphy=9010811&hvtargid=pla-1277450139760&psc=1&asin=0593234510&revisionId=&format=4&depth=1

Katie, Byron & Mitchell, Stephen (March 19, 2002). *Loving What Is: Four Questions That Can Change Your Life.* Three Rivers Press. Retrieved from, https://www.amazon.com/Loving-What-Four-Questions-Change/dp/0609608746/ref=tmm_hrd_swatch_0?_encoding=UTF8&qid=&sr=

Kleinplatz, Peggy & Ménard, A (March 19, 2020). *Magnificent Sex: Lessons from Extraordinary Lovers.* Routledge Publishing.

https://www.amazon.com/Magnificent-Sex-Lessons-Extraordinary-Lovers/dp/0367181371/ref=sr_1_1?crid=36QQ15Y113HZ7&keywords=Magnificent+sex&qid=1640015880&sprefix=magnificent+sex%2Caps%2C153&sr=8-1

Kornfield, Jack (2022). *RAIN: Principles for Mindful Transformation.* Retrieved from https://jackkornfield.com/doing-the-buddhas-practice/.

Lev, Avibail, PsyD & McKay, Matthew, PhD. (March 1, 2017). *Acceptance and Commitment Therapy for Couples: A Clinician's Guide to Using Mindfulness, Values, and Schema Awareness to Rebuild Relationships.* Context Press. Retrieved from https://www.amazon.com/Acceptance-Commitment-Therapy-Couples-Relationships/dp/162625480X/ref=sr_1_3?crid=1PQEZAQ4YVYRO&keywords=acceptance+and+commitment+therapy+for+couples&qid=1645454865&sprefix=acceptance+and+commitment+therapy+for+couples%2Caps%2C69&sr=8-3.

Linehan, Marsha M. (January 7, 2020). *Building a Life Worth Living: A Memoir.* Random House. Retrieved from https://www.amazon.com/Building-Life-Worth-Living-Memoir/dp/0812994612/ref=tmm_hrd_swatch_0?_encoding=UTF8&qid=1652878648&sr=8-4.

Lynch, Thomas R., PhD FBPsS (February 15, 2018*). Radically Open Dialectical Behavior Therapy: Theory and Practice for Treating Disorders of Overcontrol.* Context Press. Retrieved from https://www.amazon.com/Radically-Open-Dialectical-Behavior-Therapy/dp/1626259283?asin=1626259283&revisionId=&format=4&depth=1

Malone, Patrick Thomas & Malone, Thomas Patrick (October 1, 1992). *Windows of Experience: Moving Beyond Recovery to Wholeness.*

Simon & Schuster. Retrieved from https://www.amazon.com/Windows-Experience-Moving-Recovery-Wholeness/dp/0671767070/ref=sr_1_1?crid=2RVKM29I94U4S&keywords=The+Windows+of+Experience%3A+Moving+Beyond+Recovery+to+Wholeness&qid=1642696372&sprefix=the+windows+of+experience+moving+beyond+recovery+to+wholeness%2Caps%2C58&sr=8-1

Mindful Staff (January 11, 2017). *"John Kabat-Zinn: Defining Mindfulness."* Mindful. Retrieved from https://www.mindful.org/jon-kabat-zinn-defining-mindfulness/#:~:text=The%20Definition%20of%20Mindfulness%3A,self%2Dunderstanding%20and%20wisdom.%E2%80%9D

Nagoski, Emily (March 2, 2021). *Come As You Are: The Surprising New Science That Will Transform Your Sex Life.* Simon & Schuster. Retrieved from https://www.amazon.com/Come-You-Are-Surprising-Transform/dp/1982165316/ref=sr_1_1?crid=57WKLTMGA2DD&keywords=come+as+you+are+by+emily+nagoski%2C+ph.d&qid=1642701525&sprefix=come+as+you+are%2Caps%2C84&sr=8-1

Nickerson, Charlotte (November 15, 2021). *The Yerkes-Dodson Law and Performance.* Simply Psychology. Retrieved from https://www.simplypsychology.org/what-is-the-yerkes-dodson-law.html

Oprah's Lifeclass (May 26, 2000). *"Does Your Face Light Up?"* Oprah Winfrey Network. Retrieved from https://www.youtube.com/watch?v=9Jw0Fu8nhOc.

RAINN (Rape, Abuse & Incest National Network). *Children and Teens: Statistics.* Retrieved from https://www.rainn.org/statistics/children-and-teens.

Rosen, Christine (Spring, 2008). *The Myth of Multi-Tasking.* The New Atlantis. Retrieved from https://www.thenewatlantis.com/publications/the-myth-of-multitasking

Stanford Encyclopedia of Philosophy (April 10, 2018). *Stoicism.* Retrieved from https://plato.stanford.edu/entries/stoicism/.

Sternberg, R. J. (1986). *A Triangular Theory of Love. Psychological Review, 93*(2). Retrieved from https://doi.org/10.1037/0033-295X.93.2.119.

Stoeber, J., Harvey, L.N. *Multidimensional Sexual Perfectionism and Female Sexual Function: A Longitudinal Investigation. Archives of Sexual Behavior* (2016). https://doi.org/10.1007/s10508-016-0721-7

Szuchman, Paula & Anderson, Jenny (June 12, 2012). *It's Not You, It's the Dishes: How to Minimize Conflict and Maximize Happiness in Your Relationship.* Random House. Retrieved from https://www.amazon.com/Its-Dishes-originally-published-Spousonomics/dp/0385343957/ref=sr_1_1?crid=1TB6CNIRCUMOZ&keywords=Spousonomics%3A+Using+Economics+to+Master+Love%2C+Marriage%2C+and+Dirty+Dishes&qid=1642695552&sprefix=spousonomics+using+economics+to+master+love%2C+marriage%2C+and+dirty+dishes%2Caps%2C67&sr=8-1&asin=0385343957&revisionId=&format=4&depth=1

Tedeschei, Richard G. (July–August, 2020). *Growth After Trauma.* Harvard Business Review. Retrieved from https://hbr.org/2020/07/growth-after-trauma.

The Work of Byron Katie. *Whose Business Are You In?* At Home with BK on Zoom. Retrieved from https://thework.com/2006/09/whose-business-are-you-minding/

Volpe, Joseph S. Ph.D. (2020). *Trauma Response Profile: An Afternoon with Dr. Albert Ellis, Esteemed Member of the Academy's Board of Scientific and Professional Advisors.* American Academy of Experts in Traumatic Stress. Retrieved from https://www.aaets.org/traumatic-stress-library/trauma-response-profile-an-afternoon-with-dr-albert-ellis-esteemed-member-of-the-academys-board-of-scientific-and-professional-advisors.

Made in the USA
Columbia, SC
25 January 2023